KA SUTURE

Ruth.,

Thanx for the doggy
play dates! Enjoy!

Susan
aka Becca

KAMA SUTURE

LOVE
IN THE TIME
OF STITCHES,
SCARS,
AND SURGERY

BY **BECCA HAUSSMANN** AND **BAE BLISS**

ILLUSTRATED BY
L.M. FISCHER

atmosphere press

TABLE OF **CONTENTS**

To the original eight:

April, Laurie, Margo, Nancy, Suanne,
Susan, Stephanie, and Victoria

WHY Kama Suture?

What is desire? An incredible drive,
The compelling force that confirms we're alive.
Why, when the body doesn't feel well,
Is the spirit of Eros as willing as hell?
A knee that is twisted, or strained shoulder blade,
We never stop trying, it seems, to get laid.
So, we boldly tackle our predicament now—
Not when to have it, but literally, how.
Kama Sutra teaches congress for limbs that still bend.
Kama Suture's for the rest of us, with parts on the mend.

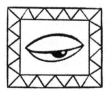

INTRODUCTION

This book is intended to be a drugless pain reliever and to provide practical information as an educational service. The goal is to demystify intimacy after surgery. It is not intended to substitute for medical advice from a physician.

Once those amazing pain medications that were sent home with us start to wear off—and when eyeing the bottom of the pill bottle causes panic—we may be looking for how *else* to feel good, now that the pharma solution is no longer an option. Oh, yes—congress!

Kama Suture developed out of a girlfriends' weekend (for eight) by the sea. One woman who recently had hip surgery was planning an upcoming rendezvous with an old crush from out of town. We brainstormed how to plan and carry out the first romantic encounter with her previously platonic friend. We all weighed in regarding our own age-related issues, with increasing hilarity. Voila! Kama Suture was born.

The classic translation of the Kama Sutra lacks advice about what to do after surgery. Surgery happens for many reasons, at all ages, when for many, the desire for romance has not waned.

How should congress be altered to accommodate the

titanium hip, the healing bone, or the post-cancer body? Kama Suture is a look at love and desire after surgery. The fifty-plus human-interest accounts in this book show how ordinary people managed congress, or the lack thereof, while keeping themselves comfortable and pain-free.

This book is for everyone who has congress, wants to have congress, or dreams about congress they've already had or wish to have, whether they've had surgery or not. Surprisingly, many adults have never gone under the knife. There is even a chapter for them. Whether you are a bored housewife, divorcé, married man, single guy, widow, or Match.com queen, this book has it all.

Based on interviews with friends and acquaintances in the Bay Area and beyond, the authors have spoken with dozens of people to understand how their romantic lives changed to accommodate their recovery and post-surgery bodies.

Reduced range of motion? Unsightly scars? In-continence while sneezing? Incontinence while doing anything? Bionic men and women with steel body parts and scarred skin enjoy healthy conjugating with a sense of humor and realistic expectations.

Whether a Millennial, Gen X-er, Zoomer, Boomer, Pre-boomer, or an as-yet-unnamed generation, anyone can learn a thing or two. You'll see in chapter two that hip surgery is not just for the oldsters of the world.

Not athletic enough to achieve some of the 4th-century manual's contortionist positions, our subjects tell their secrets as to how they keep on keepin' on. So, get out the K-Y jelly and get ready for some blow by blow accounts of how to Kama Suture. As "to Google" became a 21st-century verb, so too, shall to Kama Suture become an infinitive of infinite possibilities in the bedroom, tales that will keep the reader in stitches from beginning to its happy ending.

Thanks to everyone who sacrificed their time to complete field studies for this book. You know who you are. Names have been changed to protect the folks who shared their stories.

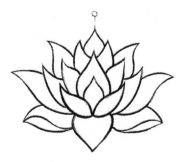

CHAPTER 1

WHAT IS THE

Kama Sutra?

The Kama Sutra, a seventeen-hundred-year-old manual on love, congress, and pleasure, as well as Indian social customs regarding marriage, was written by Mallanaga Vatsyayana in 300 A.D. and translated in 1883 by Sir Richard Francis Burton, an explorer, world traveler, translator, and orientalist. Burton was an accomplished man with a sixteen-page Wikipedia entry. His translation of the Kama Sutra is a treasure trove of the sexual do's and do-nots of the 4th century, complete with lists of whom to do and whom not to do.

In the translation of the Kama Sutra, a man with many wives is shown in an illustration satisfying six women at once, two with his fingers, two with his toes, one with his tongue, and the last with his lingham. 21st-century guys have it easy since it is culturally desirable to focus on one woman at a time. That takes the pressure off, doesn't it?

The Kama Sutra is only 20% about congress and 80% on how to live well and have relationships. This book is 100% about getting back to congress after stitches, scars, and surgeries, and most but not all of those interviewed in this book are in long-term monogamous relationships.

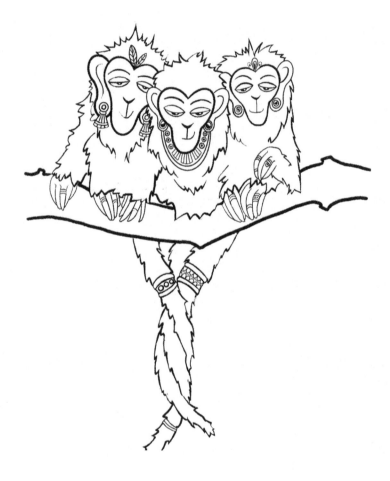

CHAPTER 2
HIPS

"If you rest, you rust."
– Helen Hayes

Whether you're a hippie or a hipster, hips are crucial in the game of love. Imagine not being able to use one of them because of the pain. Roxanne was too young to give up congress, plus she wanted kids. Robert, the roadie, could finally afford to get it done.

Senior Surgery at Twenty-nine

When most people think of hip replacement, they think of a sixty-something ex-athlete who needs a retread. Roxanne was thirty-nine when she had her second hip replacement surgery. She had fallen off a horse at the age of thirteen, and although the doctors treated her broken arm, they missed her injured hip.

In tenth grade, when Roxanne tried out for cheerleading, her friends made the squad, but she didn't get picked. When she could no longer swing her leg up and over the bar of a boy's bike in eleventh grade, she wondered why but didn't do anything about it. After all, she was in high school and had bigger fish to fry, like boys, going to prom, graduating, and getting into college.

After marrying Dan, a skier, at the age of twenty-three, she discovered she hated skiing. It made her groin hurt, a lot. She had an x-ray and was told she'd someday need a hip replacement, as in thirty years in the future. But becoming pregnant three years later showed Roxanne how serious her bad hip was affecting her life. She could only swim for exercise because it just hurt too much to do anything else.

During congress, Roxanne couldn't bend the leg with the sore hip. She could only do it standing up with her husband behind her, her left leg remaining straight to stay pain-free. She and Dan were unknowingly following the position—congress of the cow. Talk about a limit of positions. They couldn't even kiss.

When she gave birth to a healthy baby girl, Roxanne couldn't put her feet in the stirrups to push. One foot went in, and the other foot had to be supported completely straight. It's a wonder she didn't poke out the doctor's eyes with her toenails.

When her baby was two, Roxanne couldn't put off the surgery any longer. In those days, the surgeon made a ten-inch incision to cut off the top of the femur bone. Roxanne was in the hospital for five days and used a walker for the next six weeks. She graduated to crutches and then a cane, but it was a long recovery. Her toddler didn't have the terrible two's, maybe because she could feel that her mom didn't need any of the added stress.

After recovery, Roxanne had good hip rotation for the first time in fifteen years, but the doctors said she wouldn't be able to carry another pregnancy. Determined to have a second child, she got the hip surgeon to agree that it would be okay if she waited at least six months post-op before trying to conceive. With newfound hip rotation freedom in her left leg, Roxanne and Dan were able to try all kinds of new and exciting positions. One of them must've made her extra fertile because she became pregnant at the six-month mark. Roxanne promised her OB that she would gain very little weight and take it easy—as much as possible with a three-year-old daughter.

At the age of thirty-one, Roxanne had an emergency C-section to welcome her second, albeit sideways-in-the-womb, healthy daughter into the world. Ironically, now that she could've put her feet into those stirrups, there was no need for it.

Ten years later, the ball at the top of Roxanne's femur bone of the horse-injured leg was popping out of the socket again. The surgeons went in again to replace same with same. Her husband was sitting in the waiting room when a prosthesis rep showed up and announced, "I'm here with the smaller ball!" The surgeon had requested it be delivered so that he could take out the bigger one and put in the smaller one so Roxanne could get better range of motion.

Now fourteen years into her second ball and socket, Roxanne no longer downhill skis, plays soccer or tennis, but she can hike, swim, bike. She and Dan can have all the congress they want with bended legs, such as the rising position. And best of all, now they can kiss.

Shine On, Harvest Moon

The week before Halloween, the Blackhawk Plaza in San Francisco East Bay sponsored the band *Foreverland* to play on a Friday night to bring business to the shopping center. Many of the singles' club members came to hear the Michael Jackson tribute band, some in costume, others not. After an enjoyable ninety minutes of dancing under the moonlight, the group gathered round to chat while the roadies took down the band equipment. One such roadie struck up a conversation, and somehow it turned to surgery. Robert was proud of the fact that he'd just had hip surgery, and he felt like a new man.

"It's all because of Obamacare," he said. "I couldn't afford it for twenty years, so I had twenty years of hip pain."

"And now?" we asked.

"I feel fifty-four years young!" he said. "I'm doing the other one next spring."

"Why so soon?"

"Well, for twenty years I favored the bad hip, so I wore out the other hip," he said. "Besides, if a Republican gets into the Oval Office, then it's bye-bye Obamacare."

"Oh, I get it, do it while it's free."

"Exactly."

One of the guys asked about Robert's scar, wondering if he'd had the hip done with laparoscopy.

"It's not too bad," Robert said, as he began unbuckling his belt.

We all froze while we watched the man disrobe.

"See?" he said. "Just a few inches."

We looked at his exposed butt cheek under the full

moon. The scar looked like a backwards "L," a few inches long on both legs of the letter.

Robert zipped up his pants and got back to work winding speaker cords.

We looked at one another.

"That's what you get for asking," I said.

"Yes," someone in the group said. "It was a double moon tonight."

Robert, with the posterior hip replacement, preferred his partner to do woman acting the part of a man so that he could lie on the bed and his scar wouldn't show (see **cowgirl position**).

P.S. A few years later, we ran into Robert at another *Foreverland* concert. There he was at the sound board. The sound check was completed two hours before show time, so we walked up and re-introduced ourselves.

Not only had Robert had the other hip done with Obama Care insurance, but he also had two back surgeries, shoulder surgery twice, and the deviated septum in his nose fixed to help with his **sleep apnea**. With no more CPAP machine to worry about, Robert can sleep better—and do other things better in his bed, as well.

Thanks, Obama.

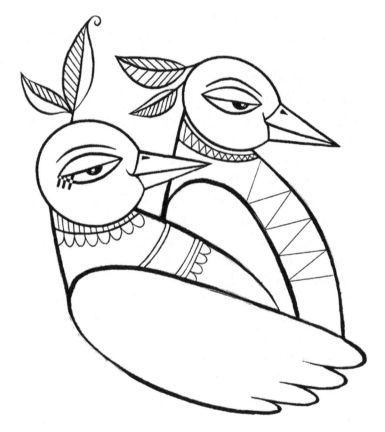

CHAPTER 3
KNEES

"Sex is a part of nature. I go along with nature."
– Marilyn Monroe

Taking a knee during a sporting event is one thing, but a crushed or trick knee is quite another. It can mess with congress, especially for the guy. Luis lucked out after his accident, and Boomer became bionic, times two.

Boomer's Tricks
First Knee

Boomer was born with two trick knees. One or the other would get locked up for no reason until he couldn't move on it. Boomer learned to unlock his knees by pulling one leg up and crossing it over the other knee in a specific way. This was needed, growing up on a working farm.

Boomer had many chores. He was a busy teen. He got

to drive the tractor, pulling the digger through rows of beet crops, stopping to check for problems when the furls didn't part correctly. One day, when he was checking the digger, his knee locked until he couldn't move. Because he was on the ground under the digger, he couldn't maneuver around to unlock the joint. He had to wait for what seemed like hours until someone found him. Eventually, his father, who was working the next plot over, noticed the tractor hadn't made progress across the field. He came over and got his son out.

The trick knee problem kept Boomer out of high school basketball, so he decided to try wrestling. At 100 pounds, he could wrestle with the best of the lightweights. After years of hard work on his family farm, his body had become solid and strong.

"All I'd have to do is just squeeze them, and they would give up," Boomer said.

Fast forward five decades. Boomer had achieved surprising things for a person with trick knees. He'd become a legend among friends on his mountain bike, downhill skis, and century bike rides (100 miles). He still dealt with the joints sometimes getting out of whack and having to put them back in place himself. It was a pain, but he was used to it.

One day Boomer found himself in the office of his friend's orthopedic surgeon. Gil was there for a rotator cuff pre-surgery appointment. After talking to Dr. Blade about his own orthopedic issues, Boomer was finally convinced to correct his nagging knee problems with knee replacement surgery. Starting with the worst one first, he would see how it went, and maybe he'd fix the other one at a later date.

The procedure went well, and true to form, Boomer was up and walking the hospital halls the next day. Easy peasy. He went back to his active life. The only drawback to his surgical experience was the need to adjust intimate encounters with his wife without disturbing the binding structure of metal and bone as the knee healed. Their favored positions might have been Congress of the Crow and Woman acting the part of a Man, although Boomer stayed mum about what their favorites were.

Second Knee

When it came time to get the second knee replacement, Boomer was ready. It was back to Dr. Blade for surgery and then rehab. The second time was more painful, and rehab was more difficult. Eventually, the knee joint was well on its way to being solid again.

A few months later, Boomer was riding shotgun in a golf cart with his friend, Gil. They approached a cart-path crossing, divided by a four-foot steel post. They were coming from the direct sun and into the shade of a cypress tree. Gil didn't see the post and plowed right into it. The force of the impact jammed Boomer's knees into the plastic console.

The other two guys in the foursome pulled up in their golf cart. With everyone holding their breath, Boomer bent down, rubbed his knees for a few moments, then stepped out and stood up, waving that it was all good.

"I'm fine," Boomer announced, stepping back in the cart, ready to hit the next tee box.

Frat Boy Blues

On a bright Saturday morning, as the sun filtered through the redwoods of Marin County, Luis headed out of his driveway on his Harley Sportster. As he rounded the bottom of the driveway, his rear wheel hit a puddle of standing water. The bike slipped out from under him. Then the full weight of the bike landed on his right knee, splitting it open "like a grape squeezed between your fingers." To make things worse, dirt and gravel had become embedded in the open wound. Luis picked himself up and looked at his knee, surprised to see the kneecap protruding through the skin.

"This isn't good," he said, even though he wasn't feeling any pain yet.

Luis parked his bike and drove his car to the nearest emergency room. The front desk clerk handed him an ice pack and told him to have a seat. After an hour in the waiting room, the knee pain really started to kick in. Luis needed attention, so he took the ice pack off his knee and displayed the open wound to the other people in the room. He hoped they would see how bad the injury was and tell the nurses.

"It worked!" he exclaimed. "Many couldn't stand to look at it, and I think someone actually got sick."

In a flash, Luis found himself being examined in the treatment room by Dr. Kneelgood.

"There is a lot of soft tissue damage," the doctor said, "and because of the deeply embedded dirt and gravel, an infection has likely started."

After giving a local injection of anesthesia, the ER team swabbed and cleaned the wound with "a mesh scrubber that looked like something people use on their bathtub."

The doctor closed up the wound and sutured four spaghetti-thin tubes for drainage on various parts of his leg.

"Those were stitched in after the drugs mostly wore off," Luis said.

The doctor told Luis to take it easy and sent him home in a soft cast.

Starting his junior year of college, Luis hobbled around on crutches. But his South-American good looks—long eyelashes and wide smile—plus his good humor scored lots of attention from the campus coeds. The first weeks of school were busy on the social front, as fraternities were rushing new students with the required parties and general mixing of the genders. At a fraternity rush party, girls flirted with him and asked how his leg cast would interfere with possible romance.

"It was both good and bad," Luis said, "good, because I was getting *lots* of sympathy and attention, but bad, because I couldn't do anything about it."

Luis hadn't had a lot of experience, being Catholic and innocent. In his mind the only possible scenario for congress—if indeed the opportunity presented itself— would be the **missionary position,** that *go-to* standard act that folks everywhere learn about and the only one on the menu college kids could tolerate imagining their parents doing. Even the standard way was a tricky proposition when one was lugging around a leg cast. For the time being, any loving Luis could hope for would be kisses and hugs along with an occasional meaningful look that suggested a future post-recovery hook-up.

The situation should have improved for Luis once the

cast came off. But while his leg remained unconfined, his knee was too tender for kneeling. For weeks to come, Luis faced a long dry spell with no hope for congress.

After what seemed to be an *eternity*, through luck, fate, or happy circumstance, Luis found a lovely girlfriend, a sophisticated lass with more experience. She introduced him to a wide spectrum of Kama Sutra poses, none of which involved pressure on the knee joint. The pressure was released when they drank champagne, as Luis was introduced to her bubbly repertoire (woman acting the part of a man, congress of the crow).

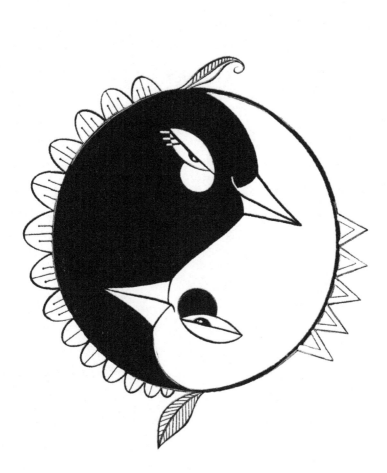

CHAPTER 4
SHOULDERS

**"Sex is the driving force on the planet. We should
embrace it, not see it as the enemy."**
– Hugh Hefner

Combining intimacy with shoulder issues takes invention
and motivation. Harvey, Danielle, and Sophie found ways
to keep congress alive while recovering from their
surgeries, with one surgery that may have saved a life.

Black Diamond Style

Harvey loved to ride his bike fast. By his mid-sixties, he
had broken the same shoulder twice during two mishaps
on steep roads. The first surgery involved grinding down
the ball joint at the top of his arm to create scar tissue to
build cartilage necessary for healing and recovery. That
part was not a surprise. But while he was awake after

surgery, the nurse came in and prepared him for a *catheter insertion*. Now, *that* was a surprise.

Wide-eyed and alert, he asked her, "What are you doing?"

"You can't risk getting up to go to the bathroom, so this will take care of it for you," she chirped.

The catheter hook-up dashed any hopes or fantasies for the other kind of hook-up that might be offered by his female friends during late-night visits.

Suffice it to say that the second accident and shoulder surgery fifteen years later involved replacing that ball joint with titanium, so that Harvey couldn't injure that area again.

Recovery after both shoulder surgeries meant Harvey had to wear a sling for weeks, keeping the arm—which was bent and rotated slightly across his torso—immobile. Since Harvey couldn't support himself with both arms, he had to take on the **subservient** position in the bedroom, as he called it. Kama Sutra calls it woman acting the part of a man.

Harvey was just as avid a skier as a cyclist. During a spontaneous black diamond race with his friends to the bottom of the slope, the experienced snowbird lost control on the mountain. As he sped up a slight rise, he was launched into the air and found himself peering down two possible landing slopes. He picked one and crashed.

Harvey broke his other shoulder, clavicle, five ribs, right wrist, right tibia and fibula, and right knee. The Tahoe Truckee emergency room was a busy place that day.

First, the doctors worked on the meniscus (knee) and set the bones in his leg. The doctors put a solid leg brace on him, since Harvey couldn't use crutches because of his broken wrist. The right wrist was also set, cast, and braced with another sling.

Harvey's movement was limited; being restricted to only kitchen and bathroom visits. With these injuries alone, congress would be possible only via the clasping position. Even the otherwise leisurely pose for lovemaking meant grand efforts of jockeying around to find the right fit, since it was his right leg, right wrist, and left shoulder that were fractured.

Harvey's final insult to injury was that he had to carry a pillow around under his arm in the sling to support and compress his chest ribs if he needed to cough. In fact, if the goal was to avoid extreme pain, any excitement like heavy breathing was out of the question until his ribs healed.

Harvey's doctors investigated a possible vascular problem and discovered a hole in his heart. While some of his former paramours may claim they already *knew* this, Harvey was completely unaware of his **congenital** condition. Ten days later he found himself in surgery again to close up the hole in his atrium. The procedure involved the placing of a blocking device there, which then stimulated tissue growth around it. It would close up the hole, a process that would take up to a year or more. Until then, the doctors cautioned him to take it easy, especially for the first month after surgery. They said no rigorous exertion or high stress, *not even the good kind*. After that initial period, congress would be permitted. But Harvey was not convinced that he had reached the safe zone. For the next two years, he remained nervous about the risk of popping the heart hole open during acts of romance. He weighed each opportunity as to whether it would be worth it, like Elaine on *Seinfeld,* who rated potential dates as sponge-worthy or not (the spermicidal sponge being a popular, single-use disposable birth control gadget during that TV show's reign in the '90s).

After getting final confirmation at the two-year mark that the heart hole was forever closed, Harvey no longer needed to channel Elaine. He was free to venture back into the arena of amor.

If he'd learned anything at all, it was that life was too short to drink bad wine. Harvey wasn't going to consume two-buck chuck when he could drink Chateau Le Fitte or Stag's Leap Cabernet Sauvignon.

Rotator Cuff Confusion

Danielle had fibromyalgia and was used to the pain that accompanied it. When she slipped and fell in Mexico, where her hotel's AC unit had dripped condensation onto the walkway between the bathroom and the kitchen, she got up and answered the phone. Only later did she realize that her shoulder was sore.

After returning to the states, Danielle was determined to fix her shoulder with exercise. She did not want surgery so she tried everything else, including cortisone shots. Two years later she could no longer lift her arm ninety degrees—it just hurt too much. An MRI showed shadowy white spider webs where her shoulder ligaments attached.

In January, Danielle told her doctor she was ready to schedule her surgery. But her ninety-six-year-old mom wasn't doing well, so she flew back to Minnesota to be with her. Her mom, Betty, was famous. Having been a flight instructor in WWII, she had a lot of friends and admirers.

People came every day to visit her and say their goodbyes. Danielle permitted twenty visitors each day on Sunday, Monday, and Tuesday. On Wednesday she put up a sign: *No Visitors Please*. People continued to knock.

"That doesn't mean me!" one intruder said. "We are good friends!"

The next day Danielle put up another sign: *Please Do Not Knock*.

Danielle had a few peaceful hours alone with her mom before she died. Her brothers hadn't come, so she had her mom all to herself.

The former Women's Air Force Service Pilot (WASP) qualified for an Arlington Cemetery burial, but Betty had wanted to be buried in her hometown of Hazelwood, Minnesota. It was no ordinary funeral. Betty had a full twenty-one-gun salute plus flyovers of various vintage airplanes that she'd flown during her reign as pilot instructor during WWII.

Danielle was the only daughter and the baby of the family, so the job of sorting and emptying her mother's house fell squarely on her aching shoulders. Danielle returned to California on April 10th and then spent the next month preparing her mother's West Coast memorial service. On May 31st she went to the WASP reunion in Sweetwater, Texas to honor her mom one last time.

Finally, in June, Danielle could focus on her shoulder. Her heart condition meant an echocardiogram ahead of time, which she passed, clearing her for surgery. Dr. Wingman went in and removed the bone spurs that had formed near the deltoid muscle. He cleaned up the jagged clavicle and fixed the severed rotator cuff ligament. Danielle was instructed to hold her shoulder in a still position with the help of a sling and a rectangular pillow that kept the arm away from her body and the pressure off of her shoulder.

Danielle had already bought a super-duper deluxe adjustable bed so that she could put her body into zero gravity with no pressure anywhere on her sensitive body.

Three weeks after her surgery, at the 4th of July party, Danielle was all smiles. Was it the drugs? The absence of shoulder pain? The fact that she'd done right by her mom, and all that work was behind her?

"I'm a happy spirit," she said.

What about congress with her husband?

"If I am on the pain meds, I'm not into it. If I stop the meds, I hurt too much."

For Danielle, for now, it's absentee congress. But that's okay. Her man will wait for her. Like a good wine, she is age-worthy. What was waiting another few months when her husband had waited nine years to marry her? But that's another story.

To Spoon Or Not to Spoon

After dinner with friends, Sophie said her goodbyes and stepped outside the restaurant, missing the eighteen-inch drop-off just past the door. She fell sideways and landed on her right shoulder. While it was painful, she told herself that it wasn't that bad, that she could tough it out, and that it would resolve on its own.

Neighbors often saw Sophie shoveling dirt, moving around small equipment, and lifting heavy tools and rocks while she did work on one of the two properties she owned. The Greek beauty loved creating outdoor living spaces, gardens, and impromptu sculptures from repurposed materials. Sophie's various work-in-progress projects provided her great pleasure.

A couple of months went by and Sophie's shoulder wasn't getting better. Chores still needed to be attended to around the properties, so she adapted by using her left arm to do them.

Sophie had to sleep on her left side to avoid the pain. This wouldn't have been a problem, but her boyfriend, Spike, complained that she always had her blond hair and back to him when they cuddled. She didn't mind spooning, but he wanted to see her face. During congress, he often checked in with her, asking, "Are you okay?"

Sophie had a fierce attachment to her side of the bed. There was no convincing her to switch places to accommodate a face-to-face position.

"I was still **smudging** the bedroom with sage," she declared, sweeping her arm back and forth, "to remove the lingering negative ghost-like energy of my ex-husband. He was living somewhere else, but I felt some remaining essence in my bedroom, and I just couldn't be on that side of the bed."

Sophie called Dr. Hipswitch, the trusted surgeon who had given her a new hip years before. In a lucky turn of events, he had recently changed his specialty to shoulder surgery.

The MRI showed a major tear in Sophie's right rotator cuff, as well as a minor injury to her bicep. Dr. Hipswitch promised Sophie he would keep scarring to a minimum, just as he had with her hip.

Everything went well, including three months of

rehabilitation. After several evenings of **coitus interruptus** with her man, who would suddenly stop in the middle of the action to ask her, "Are you okay? Am I hurting you?" Sophie was able to resume face-to-face intimacy with Spike in the half-pressed and clasping positions.

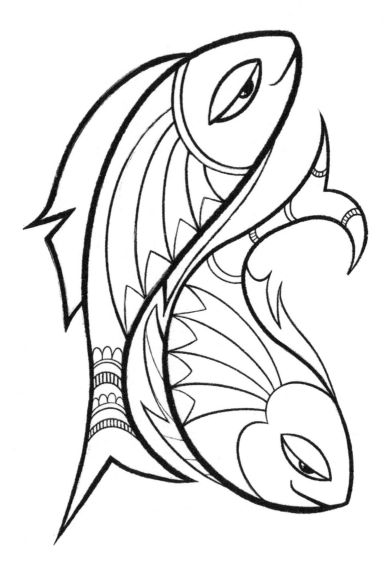

CHAPTER 5
HEAD AND NECK

**"Whoever called it necking was a
poor judge of anatomy."**
– Groucho Marx

From car accidents and bike accidents to a lifetime of neck injuries, Jolene, Boomer, and Sally had one thing in common—pain. It's hard to neck or to do anything when you have a headache.

Beauty Shop Talk

"Why did this happen to me, Doc?" Jolene asked. "The kid doesn't have a scratch."

The hairdresser had gotten into a car accident. The teenager who hit her walked away unscathed, but Jolene had disc damage to her cervical vertebrae.

"Your neck is like a glass vase, very fragile," the doctor

said. "The teenager's neck is like a piece of rubber."

Jolene went through two neck surgeries where Dr. Cuello cut through the front of the neck to get to the spine. She still worked as a hairdresser while wearing a cervical collar. She loved to quilt, sew, and style hair. Jolene did such a good job of covering up gray hairs and transforming them into beautiful fake blond tresses, she has had many years of happy clients.

Jolene's next client, Kate, a redhead pushing eighty, when asked about surgery and her love life, stated, "Well, I've never had surgery, and I'm not getting any. My gentleman friend is in his mid-seventies, and men in their mid-seventies need Viagra, you know."

Kate's boyfriend, Morty, was a challenging vintage and missing out. Kate was a red-hot octogenarian.

Jolene asked why Kate's friend didn't take Viagra, as the little ladies under the hair dryers listened and drank from their coffee mugs, but Kate wasn't dishing that day.

Jolene was almost seventy and just as active as ever, although she'd had to retire as a flight attendant ten years before. She said that congress wasn't that high on her list anymore. She was like Morty and wouldn't engage in congress.

"And if he doesn't like it, too bad!" Jolene said. "In my house, it's my way or the highway."

For Kate, Morty, Jolene, and her hubby, it was absentee congress.

Who's the Real Pain in her Neck?

Sally, a petite hospice nurse, took a gymnastics class at Cal Berkeley. As she was doing knee drops and flips on the trampoline, she landed wrong and hit her head on the springs and was knocked out for a few seconds. Someone called an ambulance, but Sally refused to go, citing that her dog, Millie, was in her car. She instead walked herself up to the university hospital.

"You're lucky you didn't break your neck," the attending staff told her.

They gave Sally a neck brace and told her to go home and rest for two weeks.

A couple of years later, Sally's car was hit broadside by a soccer mom who had run a stop sign with a carload of kids. Since it happened before car-airbag laws, Sally's head bashed against the window.

Sally also swam on a master team, so she thought the ensuing neck and back pain was from that. Over time, Sally couldn't ignore the pain. She went to the doctor and was diagnosed with three blown discs and severe stenosis, which compressed her spinal cord to a quarter of its diameter.

The doctors recommended disc removal and fusion using bone from her leg, but Sally was having none of it. She didn't want the pain and surgery of a bone graft. She allowed the surgeons to remove the bad discs, but the remaining disc structure would have to fuse naturally.

Hours later Sally woke up from the surgery with burning in her right hand. Post-op analysis concluded that her spinal cord had been nicked during the procedure and was causing the sensation. Still, Dr. Poke recommended that she go home and rest. Everything would take care of itself.

Sally and her family had booked a scuba diving trip to the tropics for the following month. Her psychiatrist husband didn't want to cancel the booking. He made calls and got permission from Sally's doctors for her to dive, so they headed to the Bahamas. After four days of diving, Sally experienced cascading waves of nerve pain extending from her chest to her stomach whenever she lowered her gaze. She knew that her condition had been exacerbated by lugging all the heavy scuba gear down to the water every day. The local medical staff offered Sally a neck brace and told her not to look down.

The old joke in medicine applies to Sally's case. The patient tells the doctor that it hurts whenever she does X, and the doctor's advice is, "Then don't do X."

Sally, unable to dive, resolved to enjoy her beach vacation by proudly donning her bikini and her neck brace for the rest of the trip.

"If there was any congress at all," Sally quipped, "it was done gingerly, with no upper body contact."

Later, a physical therapist instructed Sally to twist a towel around a doorknob and somehow hang her body from it for traction. That sparked some original poses not found in the Kama Sutra, but just as exotic.

One Kama Sutra position would be the side-by-side twining position with the help of pillows and other bolsters.

Boomer's Boomerang

Near the end of an epic mountain bike ride in Truckee, Boomer rounded a familiar corner onto his street, followed by his biking buddy, Romy. They were both part of a regular cycling group that had been riding together for decades. That day, it was just the two of them. Romy, younger and single, had long been the dream girl of the mostly male contingent.

They were rolling into the neighborhood at a fairly good clip, Boomer in front, Romy a few yards behind him.

The front end of a large white SUV suddenly appeared out of nowhere, heading into the intersection at the same time. Boomer swerved to avoid hitting the car, his rear tire skidding on loose rocks. It sent him down hard. Romy jumped off her bike and ran to help. Boomer's forehead was gushing blood. His helmet had come off.

Boomer was on blood thinners since he'd had a stroke the year before. At that time his wife, May, had found him barely conscious, crumpled facedown on the garage floor. She knew the classic signs of stroke due to her mother's history, so she rolled Boomer over on his back and asked him to smile. When he smiled crookedly, she called 911 and got him the immediate treatment he needed to fully recover and get back to riding a bike.

Now he was in trouble again. Romy took off her shirt and pressed it against the wound to contain the bleeding. She called 911 and flagged down a passerby to go to the condo and tell Boomer's wife. May rushed out to her car to go find her husband, only to learn he was at the end of their street.

Minutes later, a helicopter touched down near the scene and airlifted Boomer to the Reno Trauma Center, while May and Romy headed down the mountain by car.

The doctors stapled the large gash in Boomer's head, cleaned him up, and kept him there for three days for observation since a head wound can indicate a concussion. May kept him home for three more days just to be safe.

Romy's bloody bike shirt was tossed into the trash. It

wasn't clear who did it, as there were a couple of other folks staying at Boomer and May's condo at the time. Romy had bought it in France on a previous bike trip. When May heard that Romy wanted to salvage it, she pulled the shirt from the trash and washed the blood right out. It was as good as new, just like Boomer's head. May and Boomer had to take it easy with congress for a while.

After his experience, Boomer said he had two regrets:

1. That he hadn't looked out the bubble window of the chopper to take in the spectacular views as they glided low over the treetops of the green forest, around the peaks of the Sierras, and down into the Reno valley.

2. That he didn't get a chance to see Romy with her shirt off, since she was pressing it on his wound and blocking his view.

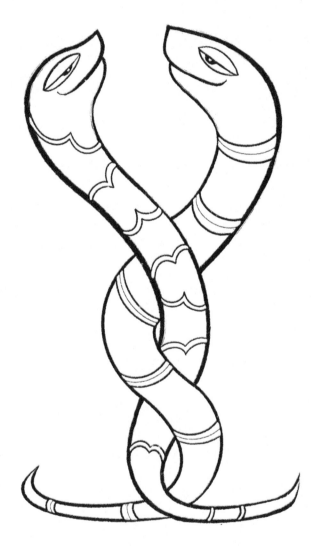

CHAPTER 6
THE BACK

"The best sex education for kids is when Daddy pats Mommy on the fanny when he comes home from work."
– William Masters

A genetic condition or a benign tumor can cause pain that creates difficulty in the love department. Both Syena and Tanya had to wait for congress and also wait for their right guy. In the end, it was so worth it.

The Short End of the Spine

"I used to be as tall as you are," Syena said about her back surgery. "I found out as a teen that I had scoliosis. I had to wear a brace throughout high school."

The girls in high school, strapped into metal devices to straighten out their spines, were on the periphery of the action, never in it. Syena had been picked on in middle school and carried a hat pin in her coat in case the girl gangs ever circled her again to tell her to stay away from a cute boy that they wanted for themselves.

"The back brace saved me," Syena explained. "My folks lived in a pretty rough neighborhood in Seattle. It was okay when my older brothers went to high school, but by the time I got there, it was filled with gangs and fighting. The girls left me alone because of the brace."

Syena didn't wear the brace to college, but the pain never stopped.

"Then I got married and carried two pregnancies, and the pain was unbearable. Finally, the doctor told me to have the surgery. I had it done when I was thirty-three. Dr. Espina fused together the vertebrae, and I lost four inches of my height. I had one more baby, so we had congress at least one more time, but eventually my ex confessed he was bisexual."

After her husband bailed to pursue his gay side, Syena had three kids to take care of by herself.

"Let's just say the whole scoliosis back thing made me stronger in more ways than one."

Syena had no congress for a long time, until the kids were out of the house. She recently met Ralph, a widower who was happy to try out many Kama Sutra positions with her, ones that she missed during those single-parent years. Like a vintage port high on the shelf, waiting to be enjoyed, Syena can be her silky seductive self with Ralph. They enjoy the packed position and the pair of tongs position.

The Aha Moment

Good-hair-day Tanya (since every day was a good hair day) was a descendent of the Blackfoot tribe from Wapanucka, Oklahoma. Her back was not so good; it hurt. Her primary care doctor sent her for an MRI. The MRI showed a most-likely benign tumor made of body fat on the base of her spine, which had grown like an octopus around her vertebrae. Although not cancerous, it was annoying and causing discomfort.

Right before Dr. Adipose made the incision into Tanya's left butt cheek, she cried out.

"Wait! Will I be able to wear a thong?"

"Yes," the doctor replied, making the incision while Tanya lay there, fully conscious with a local anesthesia.

"But I've never worn one before," she said, laughing at her bad joke.

Twenty-seven stitches later, three layers deep of nine stitches each, Tanya lay in bed, unable to move.

"I'm going on a bike ride," her husband called out on his way out the door.

A little sympathy would've been nice.

"You do that," she called back, too sore to turn over.

So much for "in sickness and in health." It was an *aha* moment in Tanya's marriage when she saw a new side of her husband. He must've been absent the day the teacher passed out the empathy card.

Tanya got divorced and had fun finding Ken doll types

on Match.com to date. So what if they were just good-time Charleys? At least she didn't have to feed, clothe, and clean up after them. She played pool with them, had fun dancing with them, and then went home by herself to her quiet little house where everyone had lots of empathy for her.

Her adult son comes and goes, but her dog, Leroy, is always there for her.

As a post script, Tanya found her new guy, Allan, on Match.com. She bought a lacey red thong, and if she accidentally drinks that third glass, they enjoy the position of Indrani.

"I look good in red," Tanya said. "After all, I am one-eighth Native American."

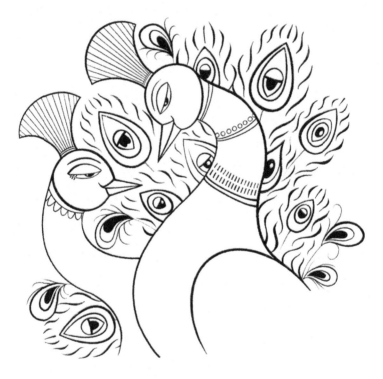

CHAPTER 7
BONES

"I'm a heroine addict. I need to have sex with women who have saved someone's life."
– Mitch Hedberg, *comedian*

Bone breaks aren't fun. They hurt a lot. Yet, after a period of recovery and rehab, the urge to merge comes back. Malcom, Kathy, Francie, Leif, and others have each found a way to deal with their broken-bone obstacles to getting back to congress.

The Butt Scootin' Boogie

Malcolm, a plain-spoken man from Big Sky country, had a serious face with azure eyes that hinted at a dry sense of humor lying just below the surface. He and his wife, Colleen, were involved in a head-on collision on a two-lane road in Northern California. Malcolm had suffered from a single-event seizure a couple of moments before the accident, had crossed the center line in their Mercury Marquis, and had veered into an oncoming truck. The truck pushed up onto their car, jamming Malcolm's left leg in the wreckage. The force shattered his hipbone socket. He suffered severe whiplash and several crushed neck vertebrae since the headrest was too low for his six-foot, four-inch frame.

Colleen received barely a scratch. The airbags had saved her. The firemen came and cut off the top of their car to get Malcolm out. He was taken by **Medevac** to the nearest trauma center some twenty miles away.

The doctors expected Malcolm's full recovery after surgery, but he was laid up for quite a while.

Dr. Spyner repaired Malcolm's C-6 vertebrate and replaced two more. He went in through the neck, with only fusion necessary.

The hip socket repair was more alarming. The doctor cut a six-inch incision in Malcolm's buttock and screwed, glued, and strapped the shattered bones back together.

"The x-ray looked bizarre," Malcolm said, "like someone went crazy with a Makita drill, sheetrock screws of various lengths, and lots of strapping tape."

After the ICU and hospital stay came weeks of rehab before Malcolm landed back home in a hospital bed for the next two and a half months. He wore a neck brace around the clock. Colleen took over Malcolm's care at home. Because he was not yet able to put weight on his left side, Malcolm was relegated to living on the ground floor while Colleen slept solo in their master suite upstairs.

Several weeks later, Malcolm was growing tired of the upstairs/downstairs sleeping arrangement. One day, when he heard his wife turn on the shower in their master bath, he hatched a scheme. He would surprise Colleen by being in their bedroom and in their bed, waiting for her when she got out of the shower. Since his early days at Air Force Academy, he'd always loved a challenge.

Malcolm made his way to the staircase. Positioning himself at the bottom stair, he sat backwards with his legs out in front of him and proceeded to hitch himself up each stair, using his upper-body strength to get him to the next step. It proved to be an arduous process to the top. Malcolm hoped that Colleen had planned a long shower (before the drought) so that he had enough time to complete the task. When he finally reached the top of the stairs, he was dismayed to realize how far down the hall the master bedroom was. He kept his eye on the prize as he dragged himself along the hallway to the bedroom and up into the bed. Grinning proudly, he lay prone as Colleen came out of the shower.

Surprised and delighted at Malcolm's determination, Colleen rewarded his efforts in the comfort of their own bed. Like an age-worthy red wine, it was worth the wait for both of them.

Malcolm enjoyed the Kama Sutra poses that involve the male on his back: congress of the crow and woman acting the part of a man.

Making Magic with a Screw and a Bone

Guido broke his left wrist three times. When he was seventeen, he broke the Scaphoid bone while playing sand volleyball at Hermosa Beach in Southern California. The doctor set the bone, but it didn't feel right.

When he was twenty-three and already on his second marriage, Guido re-broke his wrist falling at a construction site where he was working. The doctors patched him up again, but eventually Guido had trouble with fine motor skills involving his thumb. He couldn't pick up quarters off of a table with his left hand.

When he was twenty-eight, Guido slipped in the mud on Kauai at a construction site and broke his wrist again, but this time he found a better doctor who said he could fix it. Three surgeries and a steel screw later, and by using a piece of bone from Guido's hip, the surgeon got it right.

Guido is happy to report that he can now pick up coins off a hard surface and, more importantly, can pleasure himself and change hands without skipping a beat. Guido is open about congress and brags about how long he can keep the mood going. He is a fun-loving extrovert, proud of his singing voice, his dancing feet, and his hairy chest. He gets away with saying things like this with a gleam in his eye, a shoulder shrug, and a smile on his face. He's just telling it like it is.

Since he's a dancer, Guido prefers to do it to an eighty-count medium shuffle so he can get into the rhythm of it. This is the same guy who says he is dating Rosie Palm, if you know what we mean (see back matter).

Vatsyayana's love manual does not address self-pleasure, except to say that the male servants performed congress of the crow on their masters to get them ready for congress of a herd of cows.

What a Tail to Tell

Gloria broke her tailbone, the coccyx, after she slipped on a patch of ice on a winter day in Iowa. This was such a painful injury that the mere thought of *any* activity anywhere in the lower part of her body inspired an immediate face of horror. Think Van Gogh's *The Scream.*

Her doctor offered nothing about how to recover, except to use the donut cushion she was directed to sit on for the next few weeks. The donut cushion was a low-tech prize of medical equipment that had to be used all day every day, even at work. It was great snickering material for the office bullies. They jumped at every chance to highlight her indignities: at the water cooler, in the break room, and through inter-office email.

"Gloria, do you want a donut? Oh, you already have one."

Poor Gloria.

If there was ever an opportunity for congress with someone at work, it would be dashed—first by Gloria's total lack of interest (a feeling that accompanies great pain), and second by the not-so-sexy image of her carrying the inedible donut butt pillow into the office every day.

However, outside the office, the petite brunette was active on social media and online dating platforms, but she was still old school. Sitting on her donut at her laptop with a glass of her favorite Claret, Gloria enjoyed taking her time, writing to and flirting with the more appealing online prospects that kept her company at night. The men were sometimes matched up by magical algorithms. Sometimes she chose them while scrolling down the cast of locals, and occasionally she grabbed them because of the sheer gravitational pull of a gorgeous profile pic of a dude living seventy-five miles away. No potential dream date chided her about the donut.

One hunky guy, Jed, seemed promising for an in-person rendezvous, but because of her unfortunate fall Gloria decided to take advantage of the courtship and extend their virtual foreplay a bit longer, until the pain and donut were gone. At that point the best Kama Sutra position involved her receiving some gentle congress of the crow between sips of her favorite dessert wine, a sweet, supple muscat.

A double dessert is always better than a donut.

I Want my Babied Back Ribs

Clint fell, along with his mountain bike, thirty feet down a ravine near a popular trail in the Oakland hills. Another mountain biker had cut off the sixty-five-year-old cyclist. Clint landed on a rock bed on his back. Not wanting to appear weak in front of his regular riding buddies, Clint managed to climb up the ravine while carrying his bike. Then he coasted down to the parking lot to his car.

On the drive home, sitting up straight in the driver's seat, Clint decided to get checked out. He swung by the ER near his house, just in case. Thinking they might just poke and prod a little and send him home, Clint dropped his jaw when they admitted him to the hospital on the spot.

The diagnosis: Clint had fractured some ribs and punctured a lung. The doctors said he would have to stay there for four or five days.

"And to think I almost went home," Clint said.

"This is going to hurt," Dr. Payne said.

The doctors inserted a drainage tube into his side.

By then his girlfriend had arrived and was in the waiting room. Although he was glad Betsy was there, Clint hoped she wouldn't hear any screams or sobs through the wall.

Days later, Clint recovered at home. Everything was still sore. While Dr. Payne had not given any recommendations regarding congress, Clint knew there would need to be changes to his sleeping routine with his girlfriend. He couldn't lie on his back because the sheer pressure of his body weight on the back ribs was too painful. He ended up sleeping in his recliner. It was the only way he could be comfortable.

It hurt to cough, laugh, even to breathe.

Having no other options, when it came to getting it on, congress of the crow would have to suffice. Clint could rationalize the request.

"I couldn't give. I could only receive," Clint said, laughing wickedly.

Clint told Betsy this activity would make him stronger and recover faster. One wonders if his girlfriend was so easily convinced.

A Bird in the Hand

Kathy tore the tendon in her thumb when she was skiing at North Star in Lake Tahoe. Her feet went out from under her and her pole stayed put, pulling her hand backwards.

The doctors called it Game Keeper's Thumb, named after the nineteenth-century job of breaking the necks of small game animals while hunting. Kathy preferred to call it a torn UCL, or ulnar collateral ligament.

After the surgery, Kathy had a cast from elbow to thumb. She was looking at two months of recovery. Since she was off work and had so much time on her hands, she logged onto Match.com to find a suitable guy. There she met Donny, and after much online flirting, they agreed to a dinner date. Unfortunately, Kathy had to eat left-handed, and sometimes she drooled when the cup missed her mouth. Not too sexy, she thought, but Donny didn't mind. He cut her peppery meat, and they cuddled up to an earthy, full-bodied Bordeaux while he fed her bites of steak.

"When can I hold a glass of wine again?" Kathy wondered out loud.

Donny provided lots of vino, then blew her mind with new positions of congress she'd never dreamed of.

"It was a fantastic four months," she said. "He did things to me that I didn't know existed."

If there was pain in her thumb, Kathy didn't notice. But Donny had his downfalls, Kathy soon found out.

1. He was financially unstable.

2. He was a smoker (like kissing an ashtray).

3. He was jealous of everyone Kathy met or spoke with.

Then life happened. Kathy's mother passed away. Kathy had to go back East and deal with the funeral, the siblings, the finances, and the house. She stood up and gave the eulogy, in which she said that her gorgeous mother had been a flirt.

"It's an apple—tree thing," Kathy explained. "But I'm not a flirt. I'm just friendly."

At any rate, Donny wasn't emotionally there for Kathy. He didn't say the right thing or do the right thing. Her mother had died. It was a big flipping deal.

Kathy knew she had to cut him loose. Her *Fifty Shades of Grey* had been fun, but Donny was not long-term boyfriend material.

"I got my cast off just in time to secretly flip him the bird," she said.

But Donny did have his strengths. Now Kathy knows about splitting of the bamboo, fixing of a nail, and the swing.

You Say Tibia, I Say Fibula

During her recent trip to visit family in Texas, Francie looked forward to a short three-day reunion with her former beau, Kirk, which involved a connecting flight to Utah on the way back to California. A few years before, Kirk had retired and left the Bay Area to be near his adult children and grandchildren. He had kept a place in the mountains, living his dream in the remote snow country of southern Utah where he and Francie had met. Kirk had easy access to year-round activities of skiing and biking.

Francie, a decade younger than Kirk, had tons of friends in the Bay Area and couldn't see that type of life for herself. They'd connected through their shared love of skiing and other outdoor adventures. But she still enjoyed her career. While their relationship had changed over the years, their friendship remained strong, including some frisky intimate perks that they still enjoyed from time to time—**friends with benefits**.

Kirk loved extreme sports, and not ever being one to

complain about pain, had a myriad of x-rays and stitches to show for it. What Kirk failed to tell Francie before seeing her was that he had a hard cast on his left leg from a recent ski mishap. During whiteout conditions at Snow Basin, he'd dropped off a ten-foot shelf at full speed and broken his tibia in three places. It was a complicated break and was going to take some time to heal.

Their romantic possibilities together would be different. Instead of reckless abandon, it was, "Watch the leg," "Take it easy," and "Can you get me more coffee while you're up?" But, ever the optimist, Francie decided that if such carnal instincts came up, she'd be ready.

"I could always just climb on top, he wouldn't need to worry about his cast, and I wouldn't get crushed."

Old-fashioned by nature, Kirk was mum about what happened during the benefits package. Francie later explained that it was the woman acting the part of a man.

Paula Bunyan

Bilateral bunion surgery is a decision not considered lightly. It includes a six-to-eight-hour surgery, several days laid up in hospital, and six weeks of limited mobility in hard walking casts, including no driving if the right foot is involved.

Paula had inherited bunions from her mother, who had inherited them from her mother. By the time she was a young adult, walking in street shoes was painful, and she didn't like how the protruding bumps showed in her favorite flip flops and sandals.

Paula had excellent medical insurance through her

work and decided it was a good time to get the bunions removed.

Her new husband, Lou, was supportive, and better yet, available to help during the long recovery period.

Bunion surgery is a major procedure involving cutting bones. In Paula's case, the surgeon Dr. Tarsaloff cut both big toe joints and then realigned them. He also shaved off the bumpy protrusion. The surgery went well, and within ten days Paula had plaster casts that went all the way up the calf to just below the knee wrapped around each foot.

There was plenty of surface area on the casts for her friends and family to sign, decorate, and color. A friend even painted some sparkles, which glittered in the sunlight.

The orthopedic tech attached rubber pegs to the bottom of the casts, which added four inches to Paula's height, allowing her to safely walk in them without crutches, if she kept moving. The need to keep moving was so Paula could maintain balance. She looked like someone on stilts.

Paula was a public spectacle walking down the street, or at the market or in a restaurant—a nearly six-foot-tall, stiff-legged, besparkled Amazon Woman.

"It's great to be tall," Paula said. "I can see way more from up here, but the downside is that I walk like Frankenstein!"

The situation presented some challenges in the love department for the newlyweds. They were looking at six to eight weeks of a new paradigm. It was awkward, but they shared a sense of humor about it. There were some positions that worked better than others. Some could be downright dangerous to Lou because the casts were as hard as dried packed plaster can be, and heavy.

The couple's intimate connections could still involve Kama Sutra positions, but not those that could be painful for at least one of them, if not both. Fixing of the Nail, the Crab's position, or Splitting of the Bamboo were not possible.

Paula and Lou took it in stride and stuck with Congress of the Cow.

As Marilyn Monroe once said, "Don't let anyone dull your sparkle."

Broken Body, Unbroken Spirit

On New Years Day, Leif and his girlfriend, Dina, were heading up highway U.S. 50 to South Lake Tahoe. They were determined to hit the first powder of the new year. Following behind in his truck were his buddy, Joe, and his girlfriend.

Leif and Dina were nearly to the summit when a car from the opposite direction suddenly veered across the lane. There was no way to avoid the head-on collision.

Two things saved Leif and Dina's lives that day. First, they were in a three-quarter-ton pick-up truck which sat higher than most vehicles. Also, Leif did *not* have his seatbelt on. Had he been buckled in, the force of the other car, which went partially under the truck motor, lifting the transmission up under him, would have trapped him under the belt.

"I would have been cut in half," he said.

Instead, the impact of the car lifted him up and pinned him against the steering column, which bashed his face. Broken glass entered his left eye. His jaw broke in four places. Both wrists broke. His left lung collapsed. He sustained a broken left knee cap and right femur, below the hip. Massive contusions and lacerations would turn his body all colors of red, blue, and purple.

His feet were broken, the right one crushed so badly that it would take three years and several surgeries to reconstruct using bone borrowed from his right hip to fuse it together.

Dina had a broken jaw.

A Caltrans crew happened to be nearby and arrived on the scene. The guys detected a gas leak, which they foamed over to avoid fire. They called in the medical emergency response, which had to use the Jaws of Life to get Leif and Dina out of the wreckage. They were rushed to the hospital in South Lake Tahoe, where two surgeons attended to Leif. Leif spent three days on life support and six weeks in traction. His jaw was wired shut. All food was pureed and given through a straw.

His buddies came to visit. They papered the walls of his room with *Playboy* centerfolds and brought saltwater taffy, a favorite treat.

"They were cruel jokesters," Leif lamented. "They knew I couldn't act on either one of these temptations!" Gina was admitted on a separate floor and was released in a matter of days.

"Being immobilized for those weeks in the hospital was bad enough," Leif said, "but the worst part was having to move back in with my parents for a while."

During the family annual Super Bowl party, Leif's mom pureed barbequed chicken and potato salad. Leif tried to suck it through a straw, between the wires in his face. When the dentist finally unwired his jaw with the help of two adorable clinic assistants, Leif was relieved.

"What will you do first?" Dr. Molare asked.

Leif flushed. Still on crutches because of pins in his feet, he glanced over to the cute help and lifted his eyebrows twice. Leif had always been confident about his fitness, even with a broken body. He knew that someday soon, congress would be back in session.

After two full months of recovery, Leif was more than ready to resume intimacy with Dina. The meds were helpful except the anti-inflammatory ones.

"Those drugs suppress the body's inflammatory response, so certain muscles could not, shall we say, get inflamed," Leif explained.

But he and Dina stuck with it. The couple found they could enjoy congress, as long as he was flat on his back, but with absolutely no weight on his body (Woman acting the part of a Man).

Later on, Leif was able to use a folding chair made of metal that he could sit down on, which added more variety to their antics (congress of the crow).

Sure, the metal was cold, but it did the trick!

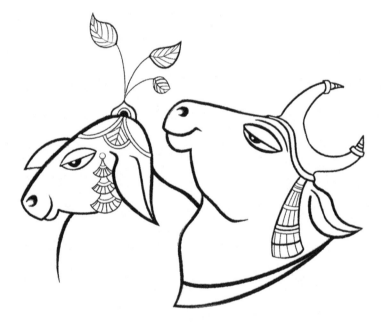

CHAPTER 8
HEART

**"I know a man who gave up smoking, drinking, sex,
and rich food. He was healthy right up to
the day he killed himself."**
– Johnny Carson

Whoever said the heart wants what it wants was right about that. Renee and Mateo followed their hearts and ended up with what they wanted, and more—Woody, not so much.

What You See is What You Get

A dancing friend was too tired to dance. His legs felt heavy. He went to the doctor, who tested him and found multiple blockages in his arteries carrying blood from the heart. After triple bypass surgery, Woody recovered and was back out on the dance floor, rocking out to his favorite seventies disco tunes. He's an R&B guy, but he'll dance to almost anything from the '70s, '80s, or '90s.

When asked if he'd talk about how it had affected his love life, Woody barked, "Why don't you come over and find out for yourself?"

Seriously, Woody? You have a girlfriend, and even though you're out on the town most nights without her, we all know she exists, and that she gets top billing on all holidays and dancing events. Maybe she's the one to ask. But, lucky for you, she seldom comes out.

Some people will open up about their after-surgery stories, and some won't. It is what it is. There is no more to tell. It was a touchy subject for Woody.

Be Still, My Heart

It began without warning. Sometimes wine was a trigger. A strange malaise would come over her. Renee could breathe, yet she was unable to take a big breath. A bone-deep ache would set in down the back of her neck and across her shoulders, making them feel heavy. Fatigue would follow. Renee, sixty and active, didn't know what was wrong. She'd had short episodes before, but after a couple of weeks of not feeling right, she went to her primary care doctor. While taking her vital signs, the doctor determined what was going on.

"You're in A-Fib," Dr. Triago declared. "You need to get yourself to the nearest ER."

Renee walked into the crowded ER lobby and was ushered into a room for evaluation. Atrial Fibrillation is an irregular heartbeat condition that can form blood clots and increase one's risk for a stroke. Dr. Corazon, the specialist there, put Renee on blood thinners and a heart rhythm medication.

The episodes continued, though they were fewer in number. Renee had to postpone a work trip because she needed to get the A-Fib under control before getting on a plane. A standard treatment to stop the episodes was to get a cardiac ablation, a minor heart procedure in which a scope is threaded up to the heart through the femoral artery. The surgeon then creates scar tissue that blocks the electrical-static circuits which cause the irregularity. The procedure was a success. The episodes stopped.

Though breakthrough episodes could still happen, Renee felt great. Then and there she decided it was time to review her bucket list. Antarctica had always been at the top of the list.

Renee was in a great relationship, but Julian wasn't interested in that kind of trip. Renee found a travel group that paired her with another solo traveler for room sharing, and her trip was booked.

A girlfriend learned of this plan and asked, "Why Antarctica?"

"If you have to ask, you'll never understand," Renee said.

Hadn't her friend seen *March of the Penguins*? Geez, it was a no-brainer.

Two months before leaving for the bottom of the world, Renee had another A-Fib episode that lasted several hours before resolving. Dr. Corazon still green-lighted the trip, saying there was a drug Renee could bring with her that could help resolve A-Fib episodes. Still, Renee felt at risk again and uncomfortable traveling with someone she didn't know. It was also a concern being so far away from emergency medical services, in case the pills didn't work. It was also possible that after taking connecting flights over many hours to reach the boat at the southern tip of Argentina, the captain could take one look at her medical paperwork and deny her access to board (they can do that).

Fast forward several years, and Renee and Julian, now married, planned their 10th anniversary trip. Jules still wasn't big on Antarctica, but after looking at other adventure trips with lots of wildlife, they found it—the Galápagos Islands! Both jazzed, they booked non-refundable flights to Ecuador and then set out to the islands to discourage any second thoughts about the trip.

From the cushy 150-passenger ship that circumvented the islands, they boarded small Zodiaks every day to access each atoll, getting up-close and personal with the wildlife specific to that place. They saw blue-footed boobies, herons, albatrosses, and huge dragon-faced iguanas which were often sprawled out across the path or street in front of them. They saw scores of colorful Sally Lightfoot crabs clinging to wet rocks where the couple swam among the Galápagos penguins. Renee checked a key item off her bucket list.

Renee and Julian walked among the giant land tortoises in the woods and meadows. The massive shells could be mistaken for gray boulders sitting there, so when the big rock started to hiss as they passed by, they knew they were too close and needed to back off.

When the male wanted to mate, he bobbed his head to attract a female. Then he bumped her with his shell to make her pull in her legs. The mating started and took several hours while the male bellowed hoarsely throughout.

Congress of the giant land tortoises is not found in the Kama Sutra. It is a puzzle to the untrained eye as to how the slow, lumbering creatures actually get the job done.

At the end of each day exploring the islands, they took the Zodiak back to the ship to drop their wetsuits and clean up. A refreshing glass of champagne or fruit punch awaited each of them back on board. It was the end of another perfect day.

Neither Julian nor Renee had injuries to rehab nor illnesses at the time, so pretty much everything was on the table as far as *congress* goes, but they were mum about their own romantic moments during their anniversary trip.

The visual of the mating giant land tortoises will have to do.

King of Hearts

Mateo was a Millennial man living his best life with John, his partner of ten years. They had resided in the windy city since his college days at Northwestern. Folks said that they were a stunning couple.

"We were happy and shared a commitment to keeping fit," Mateo said. "We worked out several times a week."

Then Mateo developed **vasculitis**, an inflammation of the blood vessels, a side effect of rheumatoid arthritis. His doctor put him on an extended regimen of steroids and told him that if he didn't follow the medication protocol, he was at increased risk of cardiovascular disease and even a heart attack. The steroids proved to be an effective treatment for Mateo's illness, but the side effects were brutal. Mateo gained 125 pounds over the next several months.

While John was a loving and committed partner through the ordeal, Mateo could sense his desire for congress was cooling off, waning with each pound that Mateo gained. It wasn't normal since John had always had a healthy libido. But he approached Mateo less frequently.

It was painful for Mateo to feel his lover pulling away, little by little. He also had to grapple with his ballooning weight gain, equivalent to adding another person to his frame. The unwanted, undeserved pounds from his medication created an increasing burden for the perfect couple.

"A fit, agile body is especially important to the physical relationship for a gay man," said Mateo.

As Mateo became more encumbered with his new body, everything physical became more difficult. Mateo experimented with new ways of having congress with John that would be less strenuous for him, hoping that introducing novelty in their love life would deepen their connection. But eventually, the relationship ended. John couldn't deal with the weight gain.

Soon after they broke up, Mateo decided to relocate to the Bay Area, leaving John and the Midwest behind. A mecca for gay culture, San Francisco was like a dream. He was struck by how open everyone was.

"West Coast people seemed more assertive, more comfortable in their own skin," he said.

Despite the painful breakup, Mateo had not lost confidence in himself. He signed onto a dating site and started meeting people.

Looking for a stable relationship and hoping for monogamy, Mateo soon found a kindred spirit in a mature man a decade older and more accepting of who Mateo was, not just a number on the scale. The relationship was solid.

On the medical front, Mateo learned he wouldn't need to continue on the steroids much longer. He had a chance to work back to the fitness level he once had. Until then, the happy couple indulged in a variety of expressions of love, including congress of the crow and lower congress.

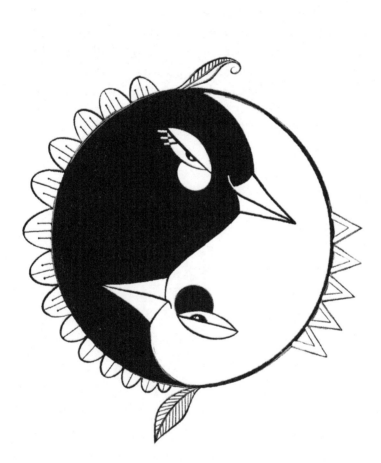

CHAPTER 9
FEMALE PARTS

**"My boyfriend and I live together, which means
we don't have sex—ever. Now that the milk is free,
we've both become lactose intolerant."**
– Margaret Cho

From complicated births and tubal ligations to menopause
and an unexpected tuchis surgery, lady parts can cause
trouble and coitus interruptus. But without the surgeries,
there'd be lots more coitus not-a-chance-us. Six women
tell how they rallied to keep their love lives intact in
whatever way they could.

Where There's a Will, There's a Way

Helen asked for a tubal ligation, a surgical procedure that
blocks the direct connection from the fallopian tubes to the
uterus. The procedure would cut off the route of the

unfertilized egg, where a bazillion sperm were swimming and waiting to pounce. She didn't want to be knocked up, yet again.

"I desperately wanted the procedure because I had produced more than enough **rug rats** running around the house, trashing the place, making demands, and draining our savings with extravagances such as food, shoes, hats, and mittens."

Helen researched the types of tubal ligations to find the most failsafe way to get it done.

Instead of the old getting-the-tubes-tied protocol, she would be getting the tubes *cut,* and then tied, which was the emerging gold standard of a failsafe plan.

Helen found the right surgeon, Dr. Clipper, to do it. Her baby daddy, Santos, loved children and could have had more, but he also loved Helen and wanted her to be happy. He agreed to the plan.

After her tubal ligation, Helen joyfully reported that spontaneous lovemaking was more frequent. "It was a relief to avoid my usual buzzkill caused by my birth control alarm system."

Helen worried that with so much carnal activity all up in there, the tubes might somehow grow back together, creating a midlife surprise. But with the added snips, she was home free.

"Who knew that surgery could introduce so many *ancient* ideas to our repertoire?"

With their newfound freedom, no Kama Sutra positions were off the table (or on it, either) for Helen and her baby daddy. A good Spanish table wine, like a Tempranillo, provided an added layer of flavor.

Ovaries, Schmo-varies

Delilah was a self-avowed health nut. She juiced, blended, and made delicious smoothies that contained all the nutrients for an active life. Yet the curly-haired beauty was plagued with persistent cysts on her ovaries. Then she found out that she carried the genetic variant which gave her a higher-than-average probability of developing ovarian cancer. Her older sister had died of the same thing a few years before.

"These are my lady parts!" she said. "They make hormones!"

Could the surgery dampen her enjoyment of congress? The good news was *no*. Her doctor prescribed hormone replacement therapy, which would keep her feminine self in balance. Since Delilah's acts of congress didn't always involve penetration, there was no worry of bumping up on surgery wounds.

Another benefit of the new hormone therapy was that it contributed to new heights of pleasure with her partner, Kat, bolstered by some lovely wine they bought to celebrate. They chose an un-oaked Chardonnay, because some Chards have too much wood.

The Sir Burton translation of the Kama Sutra has no reference to female-female pairings, but other early Hindu texts of that era indicate otherwise. We can read between the lines and assume that Delilah and Kat enjoyed congress of the crow during and beyond her recovery.

You Can Ring my Bell

As many of us know, spontaneous congress depends on adequate lubrication, something that becomes less available in aging bodies.

Rita talked to her doctor about the common problem of how to engage in congress without the first step of rifling through nightstand drawers for the flavor-of-the-month lube in a tube.

Rita asked for and got a prescription for an estrogen ring, which was placed up inside the upper third of the vaginal vault. It began dispensing that magical lube-producing hormone.

"It eliminated the need for the lube tube. I was so happy that I no longer needed to deal with that sticky yet slick substance. It got all over us both, plus the night-clothes, the bedding, and sometimes on the floor when the open tube dropped, after things escalated from frisky to freaky."

Rita couldn't wait to surprise her boyfriend with a ready, willing, and naturally lush yoni when he arrived home from a trip.

What Rita did *not* anticipate were other potential problems that resulted from rapid hormone fluctuations: an emotional roller coaster ride of irritability, sometimes violent thoughts, and tearfulness as if she were a moody teenaged girl. Any little problem that arose overwhelmed her, sending her to the end of her rope. Not knowing what was going on, Rita thought she was stressed out by life. She was turning into a hormone-fueled cyclone.

In a desperate action to achieve better mental health, Rita decided to yank the thing out by herself. It was hard to pull the ring out without the aid of the medical extraction devices. She tried and tried for days between trips to the store, going to work, and taking her mother to appointments. Every chance she could, she went home and struggled to get the sucker out. She finally managed to remove it. No harm was inflicted to tissues during the execution of the delicate maneuver (no diagram to follow).

"Within minutes, I began to feel more like myself, emotionally stable and desirable," said Rita. "And the lube in a tube worked out just fine!"

Rita and her man enjoy the mare's position while drinking a Montana red blend, aged in American oak. Neigh!!!

A Basketball Team

Deidre closed the window of her Taurus hatchback on her fourth finger and broke off the tip. No cast was needed, but boy, did it hurt! It didn't affect her love life at all.

What did affect her congress was being too fertile for her husband. He already had two boys from a previous marriage, and when she gave birth to his third child (her first), he was pleased.

"Fifteen months later, when I gave birth to his fourth son, not so much," she said.

Deidre now had two stepsons and a set of Irish twins (fifteen months apart). She stopped nursing the baby when she became pregnant again, worrying that her **alopecia** would return and she'd lose her hair.

"Too many hormones going to the babies," she said.

Her husband, Larry, now father to four boys, didn't

touch her for two years.

"The joke was that if he sneezed when I was in the same room, I'd get pregnant again. He finally gave in at the two-year mark, and our love life resumed."

"I thought I'd try for a girl by making things more acidic," Deirdre said.

She remembers using vinegar to achieve the right pH environment. Little did she know she was already pregnant. Another boy was born eight and a half months later.

Larry talked of having a vasectomy.

"The two older boys were still in diapers when my third came along," she said. "They all potty-trained together. The oldest was three and a half, the middle one was two, and the baby thought it's just what you did, to not wet your pants."

At about the same time, Deirdre's OB/GYN suggested she have a hysterectomy because of her heavy menstrual flow due to fibroid tumors. She was becoming anemic due to the lack of iron from the blood loss, the doctor told her.

"You're done having your children," Dr. Whiner said. "You don't need your uterus anymore."

"In those days, it's what you did," Deirdre said. "You didn't question the doctor. If he said you needed a hysterectomy, then you needed a hysterectomy."

All the nurses concurred with the doctor, whose word was gospel.

"It was a way to generate income for the doctor," Deirdre admitted.

It never hurts to get a second opinion. Deirdre wouldn't have dreamed of it way back then, but nowadays a woman can go see another OB/GYN and avoid an unneeded surgery. Today there are lots of female OB/GYNs.

"You don't need your pinky finger either," one female OB/GYN said. "But that doesn't mean we are going to cut it off."

Deirdre has always felt deprived of a daughter. She has lots of girlfriends, but it's not the same as having that mother/daughter bond. The good news is that she has a niece who has become like a daughter to her.

"I felt shafted by the doctor who insisted I have a hysterectomy."

As for congress, Deirdre never seems to have trouble finding it when she needs it. A friends-with-benefits arrangement with a younger man works out well for the mother of five adult sons. Just like her younger man, she prefers a young blush wine that doesn't require a lot of aging while they enjoy the pressed position.

A Pain in the Butt

Kelly needed a rectocele operation a few years after giving birth to a daughter.

"I'd never heard of it," she said, "until I needed to have one. There are a million types of surgeries out there."

Kelly had a baby at forty-six years old, and it wasn't until she was fifty-two that she needed the surgery. She'd had pain for a few months and felt like she had holes in her rectum. The sensation of not feeling able to complete a full bowel movement was another symptom. Her OB/GYN at Alta Bates in Berkeley recommended surgery.

"My baby, Lily, weighed just eight pounds, so I couldn't believe the vaginal delivery caused this to happen to me."

Rectocele is a tear that happens in the wall between the vagina and rectum when the rectal tissue bulges through this tear and into the vagina as a hernia.

Kelly's recovery period involved **Sitz** baths, a plastic donut ring to sit on, and time to heal with absolutely no congress. After that, Kelly had to use healing massage creams to help make her openings flexible again since the scar tissue that formed after the surgery was not flexible.

"I had ten stitches in my **tuchis**," Kelly said.

Kelly had split with her baby daddy by then, so there was no chance of a good sleep-over to complicate recovery, but a split of zinfandel and 70% cacao dark chocolate kept her warm and happy.

All we can say is, Kelly, we're glad you're over this. What a pain in the butt.

The Unkindest Cut of All

Olivia was looking forward to the birth of her first child, but she was *not* looking forward to the hours of excruciating contractions during labor. Being a nurse in Berkeley, Olivia had been through labor in action and experienced the natural process of relentless contractions necessary to send it out of the uterus and down through the vagina.

"Baby—good," she said, "vagina—traumatized."

Adorable and wondrous new baby aside, the utter carnage left behind in the birth canal was enough to make her want to swear off congress and childbirth for the rest of her life. Her husband agreed when he stayed to watch.

"It's amazing that people ever decide to have more

than one kid," Olivia said.

Her second time at bat, Olivia hoped nothing would come out of left field. Olivia's OB/GYN, Dr. Bush, realized that her second baby was in the **breech** position. Even after being successfully flipped by the medical team (an **ECV**—an **external cephalic version**—a series of intense, uncomfortable massages onto the uterus and fetus), the little guy flipped right back. Was it a foreshadowing of the future rebellious teenager, perhaps? It looked as if the baby would not be able to come out the old-fashioned way.

Olivia needed a caesarian section, a surgical procedure where the baby is lifted out of the womb through an incision in the mother's abdomen. No labor, no pushing. The vital young woman, whose healthy lust for congress had sharply increased with spiking pregnancy hormones, was happy to know that her yoni would remain calm and undisturbed. She imagined she would avoid the vaginal recovery period that others had to endure and could resume congress sooner. However, it was not to be. Dr. Bush cautioned that there should be no carnal activity for at least two weeks. After all, there were stitches and an incision involved. Only then would yoni and lingham be able to join in congress without complication.

Olivia and her equally congress-starved husband waited just five days, then caved and decided to go for it. They commenced with such passion, such white-hot fervor, a scenario of such raw pent-up desire, that it was something which could only be expressed in a **bodice-ripper** novel. They couldn't get going fast enough. But soon there was a problem, some sort of barrier at the site. Nothing was getting through.

Olivia and her husband untangled arms and legs to unravel the mystery. Nothing serious was wrong. It was just a strip of pink nylon. During all the hasty fumbling, they had forgotten to remove her panties. The pair celebrated with an assertive pinot noir wine, containing notes of ripe cherry, after enjoying the twining position.

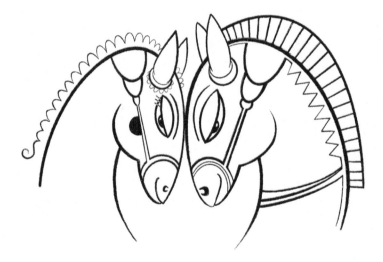

CHAPTER 10
MALE PARTS

**"Women need a reason to have sex.
Men just need a place."**
– Billy Crystal

Being snipped down there is a terrifying prospect for most guys. To avoid it, they either end up with more children or the wrath of their wives/partners. If they do get it done, they are supposed to go back to get the all-clear (no more swimmers) from their doctor. Hernias aren't much fun, either. See below.

Shooting Blanks, or Not?

When Ed realized that the seed that sprang from him every time he had congress was the reason that his wife's pregnancies soon followed, he knew he had to do something. His doctor confirmed that, yes, babies *could* indeed result from a robust emission of the swimmer seeds into a fertile yoni. Dr. Bohner suggested that Ed have a vasectomy.

"When I learned what would happen," Ed said, "when, and with what—such a sharp cold instrument snipping around close to my manhood—I was terrified."

With some panicky back-pedaling, Ed postponed the surgery until a more compelling argument came from his wife.

"Nothing shall happen in the bedroom until the deed is done," she said.

After Ed had the procedure, there was no forthcoming medical advice from Dr. Bohner about congress. There would be a follow-up visit scheduled involving a small cup for Ed to fill.

"Unfortunately, no picture magazines were offered to help me achieve the goal," Ed said.

Ed's full cup would be tested to make sure that *none* of the little buggers had made it through and were swimming around in there. In other words, had the vasectomy worked?

"I never did do the cup thing," Ed admitted.

Maybe Ed didn't want to face his ultimate betrayal of his body's teaming fertility. Or perhaps it was simply the absence of said reading materials.

In any event, it was Russian roulette for Ed and his wife from then on, celebrated with a bottle of splendid Syrah from their extensive wine cellar (the old nursery).

Hopefully they kept the crib and baby stuff.

I've Got This, Honey

Sledge ran a tire shop and was used to hard work and pain at the end of the day. What he wasn't used to was the pain he'd endure by agreeing to have a vasectomy.

Sledge's wife, Judy, had given birth and then decided to stop taking the pill. Then she had an accidental tubal pregnancy. The OB/GYN figured out why she was in so much pain.

"Judy," Dr. Ovo said, "if this tubal pregnancy happens again, it could kill you. Since you don't want more children, you need to get your tubes tied."

Sledge, the macho guy that he was, told Judy not to worry or have the surgery.

"I'll take care of it," he said.

A vasectomy would be a much less invasive procedure with a shorter recovery time. But after his urologist, Dr. Snippet, made the first cut, Sledge wasn't feeling macho anymore. The way he was sweating and grimacing prompted the doctor to ask him, "Do you want me to stop, and you can come back later to do the other side?"

"No!" Sledge said. "I don't ever want to do anything like this again. Just get it done!"

That was Friday morning. By Friday afternoon, Sledge was back at his tire shop working away. On Saturday, he worked a half-day at the shop, and on Sunday, he was finally able to sit down and recover.

Sledge had to return with a sample of his sperm after so many protected acts of congress to make sure the vasectomy had done the trick. He worked it into his tire shop schedule, after a particular female customer in her tight sweater and skirt brought in her car for repair. After she left, Sledge went into the bathroom and, with the image of the sweater girl in mind, filled the cup and took it to the doctor's office. Dr. Snippet tested the contents and said Sledge was good to go.

Later that evening, Sledge told Judy they were now safe to have all the congress they wanted without the risks of getting her pregnant again.

"What do you mean you took a sample in?" Judy asked. "Where did you get it? How did you get it?"

Sledge had to chuckle. It had never occurred to his wife that he could do it on his own, without her. He never told her about the sweater girl.

"I took care of it," Sledge said as he popped the cork of a luscious Moscato.

And he did.

The Double-Double

Never-been-married Bruce was halfway through a years-long relationship with a divorced mom of four when he saw his physician regarding two bulging **inguinal hernias**. He attributed them to heavy workouts at the gym.

Dr. Deekupsie explained that he could have the elective surgery right away or wait until things got **ischemic**.

"Then you'd have to go in for emergency surgery," she said.

The matching bulges in Bruce's abdomen wall didn't hurt at all.

"The idea of my abdominal muscles, collapsing and squeezing to death the protruding sections of intestine, seemed nothing to look forward to," Bruce said.

Bruce didn't waste any time.

"I don't want the **ischemic** thing," he said. "Let's do the surgery."

On the scheduled Monday morning, Bruce's girlfriend, Katarina, drove him to his 7:00 A.M. pre-op appointment. She waited the two hours during the outpatient procedure and then drove him home after recovery. He went to bed and slept. She stayed there to watch over him.

When Bruce needed to pee, he tried to get up and realized that every movement hurt— to sit, to stand, to walk.

"They used staples when they put the mesh over the holes in the abdominal wall to keep the intestines inside where they belong. The surgery invaded my core muscles," he said. "You use your core muscles for everything."

Bruce didn't have matching scars since the doctor went in through the belly button. He had two weeks' recovery time of no congress.

"I wasn't physically strong enough to do it until then."

There was another concern.

"The doctor told me that my penis might turn black and blue but not to worry about it. How could I not worry? But it didn't."

As for the relationship with Katarina, the mom of four, it didn't last.

"She was a good Catholic girl, and as you know, I am the anti-Christ. I want religion to go away. Teaching kids that the Earth is only 6000 years old is child abuse."

Bruce is a STEM guy: science, technology, engineering, and math. He's an atheist and proud of it.

"Human beings behave so freaking badly," he said.

"One of the main reasons they behave badly is in the name of religion. Look at the guys who flew an airplane into a building."

Still, he felt bad that he couldn't make it work with Katarina.

"She couldn't let go of her lifelong beliefs," he said. "I remember telling her she was a great girlfriend except for the Jesus thing."

Bruce had **absentee congress.**

Hernias and Hotties

Jeremy often flashed an impish grin, leaving one to think he had just gotten away with something and that he was as pleased with himself as the Cheshire cat. But he wasn't smiling when, after a day of heavy yard work, he felt a bulge in his abdomen near his groin. He called Rachel, his fiancé, in Lake Tahoe, 180 miles away. She told him to call the doctor.

They had been together for a few years, living in separate states, the arrangement being that they remained in their respective homes, his in the East Bay. One would stay with the other for a few days or weeks. Mostly, it was Jeremy hopping on the fifty-minute Southwest flight from OAK to RNO and back.

Jeremy had more control of his schedule as a business owner. In fact, it was rare that Rachel came and stayed at Jeremy's, though he had a spacious home. She couldn't get away from her family business. During his visits, Jeremy was an ally and sounding board for Rachel when it came to her own business concerns, worries, and responsibilities. He was a true partner.

Then the doctor told him the news.

"You have an **inguinal hernia**," said Dr. Bellagio. "You'll need to get that fixed."

The hernia repair surgery in his groin area, inches away from you-know-what, was not going to be fun. Jeremy tended to look for the good things that come out of the bad.

"I was lucky that at least the person with the scalpel was a hot female doctor," said Jeremy. "She was so cute, so I thought there was no way she could hurt me."

Jeremy knew this attraction to Dr. Hotlips would foster some unsettled feelings. Given the location of the incision, he was embarrassed that his private parts would be on full display.

After his outpatient surgery, Jeremy's neighbor drove him home, as morphine circulated through his body. He was feeling no pain. In fact, later that afternoon, still on his morphine high, Jeremy decided to go outside and water his shrubs in 104-degree temperatures.

The next day, it hit him. Jeremy was dehydrated from both the drugs and from sweating in the garden during the heatwave the night before. His incision hurt. He wanted a beer, so he threw caution to the wind and decided to drive to the store for a six-pack. Jeremy drove the half-mile down the hill to the intersection with the stoplight. It was red.

"The next thing I heard was the car behind me honking, because the light had turned green. But I was so spaced-out from the pain meds that I forgot to drive."

Jeremy's brain finally kicked in and he turned the car around and slowly headed back home, with no beer.

When Jeremy's bursting bladder signaled a bathroom run at night, he couldn't get out of the overstuffed bed. He couldn't use his stomach muscles or even roll over.

"It was a real bitch to get up or bend over," he said.

The logistical problem of getting to the loo persisted until Jeremy rigged a rope around the doorknob. Now he could pull himself up and climb out of the pillow-top-mattress bed.

The possibility of any type of congress seemed remote, and Jeremy said there was no way he would ask Dr. Hotlips about it. He didn't want to hear that he'd be useless for at least three weeks.

"No man needs to hear this anyway, especially from a hot surgeon!"

Jeremy's fiancé, Rachel, was unwilling to make the three-plus hour drive to give Jeremy some TLC during the initial post-op days. He had to manage by himself.

Enforced celibacy for Jeremy led him back to considering his pledge to his girlfriend. Going through it all alone, he began to question Rachel's true commitment to him and to his well-being.

"Rachel seemed to have no time to care for the so-called number one person in her life—me!"

After a thoughtful review of their relationship over the next several weeks, Jeremy decided he deserved something better. He was looking for a vintner's select reserve.

Single again, Jeremy's Cheshire grin and happy nature pulled many gals into his orbit. The next time, he made sure the love of his life kept him a priority, both in sickness and in health.

He is now married to Deb and living the dream.

A Missed Pit Stop

Sergio, a bearded hippie, had multiple surgeries: one on his shoulder, the second to remove a skin cancer, and the third for an **inguinal hernia** that the doctor described as particularly humongous. After the hernia surgery, Sergio waited the appropriate six weeks before going for a test drive to see if everything still worked right.

Sergio got his engine started with his wife, but as congress began, he panicked.

"What if there'd be water mixed with the oil?" he asked.

As we said, the hernia had been a whopper. He was worried there would be blood in his semen.

In the middle of the first few laps of foreplay, Sergio decided to forfeit the race. Instead of pulling into the pit, he bypassed it completely and headed to the bathroom. It was definitely time for the oil to be changed, so he did it in the sink, and sure enough, there was water in the oil as he had feared. Sergio decided to rest up a few more weeks before he took his race car back around the track.

The first time he drove his real car after the hernia surgery, Sergio swung his legs to the left to get out of the driver's seat, and as he pulled himself to a standing position, he felt a rip in his abdomen. He was sure he'd see blood all over the ground, but Dr. Bulger explained later it was the scar tissue from the surgery that he had displaced with no real consequence, other than the sensation of tearing apart his insides.

After Sergio's surgery and the six-week waiting time, he and his wife attempted congress. She took the role of woman acting the part of a man while Sergio stayed safely on the bottom. With a bad shoulder, he couldn't support his own body weight.

A good surgery provides the patient with a good story to spin for years to come. Sergio relished every moment of telling his whopper over a glass of smoky, rustic happy-hour red.

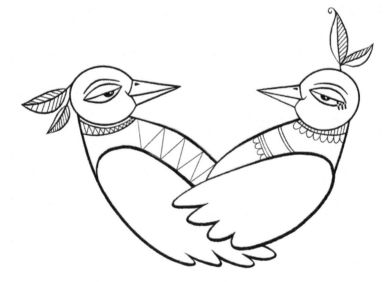

CHAPTER 11
EYES

"During sex I fantasize I'm someone else."
– Richard Lewis, *comedian*

The expression *love is blind* takes on a whole new meaning when the eyes stop working. Antonio and Darren tell how they set their sights on congress and got their mojo back.

Hollywood Good

When asked if he'd ever had any surgery, Antonio said, "Look at my face and tell me what I've had done."

Antonio had a full head of gray and white hair, deep brown eyes, a chiseled nose, and a nice smile. What had he had done? A face-lift? Botox? A nose job?

None of the above: he'd had his right eye replaced with a fake but moving one, not a glass eye. The eye was moving similarly to his other eye. Only an optometrist had noticed it didn't track the same as the left one.

"I was a little kid," he said. "I was playing with knives. My mom still feels guilty about what happened. I was cutting a cord off of a box. The knife was pointing up, and when it cut through the cord, the knife kept going and went into my eye."

At the age of four.

"There wasn't any 911 system back then," he continued. "Mom called the police. I remember riding in the police car."

Regarding the doctors—

"They saved my eye, but I only had 10% vision, and my eye had a white streak in it."

Regarding sports—

"I still did baseball and basketball. I was able to play with the one good eye."

Regarding his family—

"My younger brother, when he wanted to be really mean, called me Cyclops."

Antonio played competitive volleyball when he was in his twenties. He kept his damaged eye for twelve more years until his doctor, Dr. Vizjh in Oakland, talked him into replacing it with the **prosthesis**. All Antonio gave up was 10% vision in that eye, and he gained so much more from a better-looking appearance.

"Two-thirds of the eye is replaced with coral, which was a living organism, and it has the same level of calcium in it as bone does. The eye muscles grow around the coral and attach to it," he explained. "Then I went back a few months later and Dr. Vijzh worked on the front third of the eye, the part you see. He painted it, sculpted it, and got it just right."

Regarding the surgeon—

"My eye doctor is so good he even does Hollywood movie stars. He doesn't tell. But trust me, they're celebrities you'd know. We all love Dr. Vijzh, those of us who've let him work his magic."

Regarding drawbacks, Antonio said that he can't go to 3D movies.

"They just look shadowy and fuzzy to me."

Regarding congress, Antonio said, "If anything, it made my sex life better. I had better self-esteem because my eye looked normal again. I prefer face-to-face. There's no shadowy or fuzzy to that."

Antonio and his woman sipped sangria while experimenting with the pair of tongs, and not the ones from the ice bucket.

The Eyes Have It

Handsome Darren was married to beautiful Morgan. He knew that someday in the distant future he would need to have surgery to remove a pterygium on his right eye. A **pterygium** is a benign opaque flap of tissue that grows on the white part of the cornea. It can be caused by too much time in the sun and surf, which the blue-eyed California athlete had enjoyed throughout his life.

The growth, slow-growing and barely visible to others, could eventually start to obstruct the pupil, at which point it had to be removed. Darren's flap had gotten to that point. His time had come; the future was now. Just barely into his seventies, Darren had put it off as long as he could. Though the surgery was a common outpatient procedure,

Darren was nervous about his eye going under the knife, after which he would be required to wear a protective eye patch every night for a few weeks to protect the stitches.

Morgan drove him to the surgery center. She decided to ease his anxious mood by joking that while her man would be going in, a pirate would be coming out!

They took a seat in the outer lobby, and when Darren's name was called, he reluctantly stepped into the room where Dr. Scraper was waiting. Morgan was still reading her *Time Magazine* when Darren came out with a protruding bandage over the eye. The egg-shaped albatross would have to remain there for the next few days.

It took a minute for Darren to scan the waiting room for his wife. He had only one working eye and his depth perception was gone. Darren couldn't wear his glasses with the bandage.

As Morgan drove him home, Darren knew how careful he'd need to be during recovery. But once he graduated to wearing a sleek black eye patch that was more reminiscent of the Jolly Roger, he hoped Morgan would see him in a whole new way. His vibe would be more like a swashbuckling pirate in a fun role-play game.

Staying clear of the patch, they could act out all kinds of certain scenarios on the high seas. Mostly, though, they were a well-grounded pair and found that the lotus position was safe for the eye, and also one of their favorite yoga poses. Both being seniors, well past middle-age and dealing with stiffening joints, the couple liked to stretch their bodies in different ways. The position was the perfect marriage of fun healthful habits. *AHHHRRRR!*

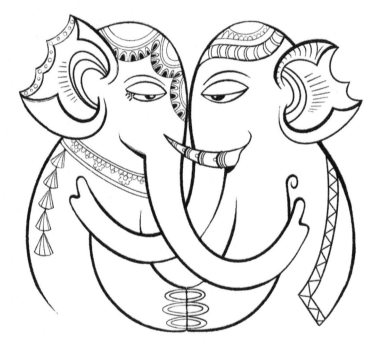

CHAPTER 12
BLOOD AND SKIN

**"Birds do it, bees do it, even educated fleas do it.
Let's do it, let's fall in love."**
– Cole Porter

Blood clots or blood infections can kill a person. So can bad burns to the skin. Red, Karli, and Sophie live to tell how they survived and also how they nailed down congress with the right or wrong guy. Plus, a nagging Becky might've saved her guy's life.

The Nightmare Before Halloween

The 911 dispatcher told Red to turn on the porch light, lock up her dog, Coco, and wait for the ambulance. It was Halloween, and Red had changed the clear bulb to a black light. Fake cobwebs framed the porch, and pumpkins lined her Tahoe duplex walkway.

Red had made dinner for herself that Saturday night and had gone to bed. A sharp pain on her right side near her ribs woke her up. She couldn't breathe. Her boyfriend, Derek, had taken her car to the Bay Area for the week where he worked. Red was home alone with no way to get to the hospital.

Her heart was racing. The paramedics pulled up to the duplex; two guys and two gals got out. One guy took her vital signs, which, he reported, were within normal ranges. His diagnosis—the twenty-year-old was fine but had panicked and worked herself into a frenzy.

"Your heart is racing, but nothing is wrong with you. You can stay here and sleep it off, or you can go into the hospital for more tests."

Red deliberated. They were saying she was fine. But she didn't feel fine, and how was she going to sleep with the pain in her side?

"Take me to the hospital," she said.

The paramedics loaded her onto a gurney and took her to Barton Memorial. They didn't bother with an IV. The hospital was just five minutes away.

"I knew my body," Red said. "I knew something was really wrong."

"Do you do drugs?" the ER doctor asked her.

"I smoke pot," she said.

"No cocaine? No heroin?"

"No, just pot," she said.

"Everything seems fine," Dr. Edwards said. "But we'll do a CT scan, just to be sure."

They administered the iodine through her newly inserted IV.

"The iodine in my body felt warm below the waist,"

Red said. "I felt like I had to pee."

Red raised her arms as instructed as she lay on the bed of the CT scanner. Her right side felt like an overstretched rubber band, ready to snap.

After she was taken back to her room, she waited for the diagnosis. The ER doctor came in, sat down, and put his hand on her knee. When he looked into her eyes, she knew it was bad news. She broke down crying.

"You have a **pulmonary embolism**," he said, "a blood clot in your lung."

"How could this happen?" Red asked.

"I see that you take birth control pills," Dr. Edwards said. "It's rare, but it can be a side effect."

Red called her mom. Her mom called her dad. Her dad called her brother. Someone called Derek.

Red was alone in the ER with no one to comfort her. She tried to sleep. At 5:00 A.M. her dad called her back. Red was beside herself.

"How could I have a blood clot?" she asked. "I'm only twenty."

"I don't know, Honey, but I can't miss any work to come see you," her dad said. "Your mom is coming."

The doctor gave Red an injection of blood thinners in her abdomen to help dissolve the clot. She would have the shots six more times before she left the hospital and then every day thereafter for a month.

They offered her Oxycontin for the pain. "No," she said.

"Are you sure?" they asked again. Red said no.

Red's friend, Chalupa, had become addicted to it and had died in a car accident not long before. The autopsy had shown both Oxycontin and Xanax in his blood. He'd run into a tree.

By Sunday morning her mom and brother had arrived in Tahoe. After a quick visit, Red's mom went to check on the dogs while Red's brother stayed with her at the hospital. Her BFF, Dallas, called crying. They'd been besties since anger management class when they were fourteen.

Her dad sent flowers but didn't come. Derek didn't come, either. Red and Derek fought over the phone. She was talking with him when the heart machine registered 180 beats per minute. She lost her hospital phone privileges after that.

Red's mom came back on Monday after taking Red's brother back to the Bay Area so that he could go to work. Her mom stayed the whole week while Red was in the hospital and the next week, too, while she recovered at home.

Back at the duplex, Red couldn't climb the stairs. It hurt to sneeze and cough. She did her breathing exercises into the breath machine. The lining of her lungs was inflamed. She had **pleurisy**.

Derek finally came to see Red after her mom left Tahoe. He cooked and took care of the dogs, but he was not consoling and had no bedside manner. At night he'd go out and leave her alone.

The blood thinner, Coumadin, which Red had to take for a full year, led her skin to bruise easily. Any cut she got would bleed and bleed.

Red got an IUD for birth control. Because she was on Coumadin, she couldn't take any aspirin or pain relievers to help with pain after the IUD was inserted. The good news was she no longer had any period at all, so there was no interruption in her romantic life.

"It still grinds my gears that the paramedics would've left me to sleep it off," Red said. "I might've died if I'd listened to the paramedics and stayed home."

Later on, to make up for his lack of visiting, Red's dad cooked her favorite dinner at his house, and served it by candlelight: pork chops with caramelized onions and applesauce.

Red had to have her blood checked once a week for a year by a hematologist. Her dad took her to UCSF to see the blood-clot gurus. They asked about her lifestyle. Their verdict—she had a higher chance of rolling over in an off-road vehicle than she did of getting another blood clot, unless...

...she led a sedentary life or became pregnant.

"Two years later, when I went to New Zealand, I had to give myself injections of blood thinners while I sat on the plane for fourteen hours."

Now twenty-seven and in the high-risk group for pregnancy, Red said, "I'm not set on having kids, but maybe..."

Red had taken a popular birth control pill made by a reputable company.

"While I was in the hospital my roommate saw a commercial for a lawyer, and she woke me up. I called right away. They got me a settlement with a gag clause."

"Derek turned out to be a jerk," she said. "We had a fight in my Jeep, and he tried to punch me, but he missed and broke the car's seat instead. He's toast."

Red has a new boyfriend, Eric, who works on a ship. He's here one month and gone the next.

"I am thankful to be alive," Red said. "I don't take anything for granted."

"I still have Coco, and a new dog, two cats, four ducks, some fish, and thirteen chickens—oh, and a garden."

The new guy floats her boat. They like the crab position and a rich Petit Verdot wine.

Wine Country Warning Signs

Karli and Jake had a wine-tasting weekend planned with friends. Friday afternoon, they drove to Karli's parents' second home in Sonora. Karli hadn't felt well that morning and had woken up with a headache, plus shooting pains in her ears. She almost passed out at work but wanted to keep their plans.

On Saturday morning she woke up in Sonora at 9:00 A.M. and felt much worse. Jake went online to Web MD to see what it could be, and when **sepsis** came up as a diagnosis, Karli disregarded it as "too far-fetched." They went ahead with their wine-tasting plans with the other couple, although Karli didn't feel well enough to participate. She slept in the car while the others did the tasting.

"I threw up in the bushes next to the winery," Karli said, "and I wasn't even drinking!"

Jake kept out a watchful eye and insisted that he take Karli to the ER while the other couple made dinner. The first ER was closed when they got there, and Jake had trouble getting the GPS to direct them to a second hospital. They finally made it to Sonora Regional Medical Center around 9:00 P.M. The clerk at the desk called for a wheelchair, and Karli was taken to a cubicle to answer questions while Jake was left in the waiting room.

The ER staff hooked Karli up to an IV and gave her fluids and painkillers. The initial diagnosis was severe dehydration from the vomiting. Jake was told she'd be released in a few hours.

At 2:00 A.M., after another set of doctors came in to ask Karli the same questions she'd already been asked six times, Karli got upset and **hyperventilated**. The nurses inserted a nose **cannula** to help with breathing.

At 3:00 A.M. Karli's diagnosis changed. Blood tests had shown renal failure; her kidneys had shut down. The desk attendant instructed Jake to go home and call Karli's parents, who were five and half hours away in Santa Cruz County.

Karli tried to sleep, but she couldn't. Her entire body hurt. The ER nurses gave her narcotics for the pain through the IV. At 6:00 A.M. blood tests showed that Karli's blood was **septic**. She was moved to the ICU for closer monitoring. The nurses helped Karli call Jake and her parents and ask them all to come to the hospital.

Karli had her blood drawn every two hours as multiple doctors and staff came through to check on her. Some thought it was a staph infection; others thought it was strep. The doctors later told her parents that they were throwing everything at the infection to see what would help. Karli doesn't remember much except for vomiting, but Jake helped fill in the blanks. He was told that her heart rate was high and her blood pressure was low. Her body was working hard with little result.

Jake, her mom, and her dad worked out a schedule so that Karli would not be alone in the ICU. Jake worked remotely from the Sonora house while Dad took the morning shift. Mom took the afternoon shift, and Jake came at 5:00 P.M. every day and spent the night there. The hospital provided a cot for him to sleep on for the eleven nights Karli was in the hospital. Karli's little brother even came up from his college in Santa Cruz to see her, and so did her best friend.

Since her kidneys weren't working, Karli wasn't urinating. Then she got pneumonia. On top of everything else, she had two respiratory therapists and daily breathing exercises to do.

Jake wasn't told much during this time. He was only the *boyfriend*, and when Karli's parents got there, the doctors spoke directly to them and ignored him. Only one ICU nurse regarded Jake with a handshake and a "good luck" when his shift ended, since he wouldn't be back for a few days.

As it turned out, Karli had **bacterial endocarditis**, where the staph infection had attached to her aortic valve, and her beating heart was sending out the infection to all of her other organs. None of the medical staff knew where the staph came from, but she had had a spider bite three years before that had become infected.

"Maybe the infection never went away and instead lay dormant until the night of May fifth," Karli said. "I had also been recently scratched by my cat."

The day Karli finally peed it was a celebration. After that, she was well enough to get out of the ICU and go back to a regular hospital room.

Karli had surgery on Mother's Day. Too much infected fluid was trapped in her hips, especially the left one. Jake had been studying for a test for promotion as an injury insurance adjustor, and he understood, since he had just learned that "hips have bad blood flow."

The doctors did an **irrigation** and **debridement** to drain the fluid and flush out the infection. Four days after her hip surgery, the doctors stuck Karli on an x-ray table and used a big needle to clean out the other hip. There are no matching scars for Karli; she is one-sided in that regard.

The doctors told Karli that if she had been older, they would've let the left hip go. She then would've had to have it replaced when the infection spread to her hip bone.

"I guess a twenty-three-year-old hip was worth saving," she said.

Karli's hips ache in the winter when it's cold or if they get too tight from inactivity due to missed trips to the gym. They also hurt when climbing up to Jake and Karli's nosebleed seats for the 49ers game, especially after walking a mile from where they park the car.

One of the doctors told Karli's parents that if Jake would've waited eight more hours to bring her in, Karli would've been in a coma by then, and it would've been too late.

"As cliché as it sounds, I know there are more important things in life than letting the small things get me down," Karli said. "The whole experience has calmed me, because you don't know when it's going to be over."

Karli's dad knew Jake was the one for his only daughter. He had gotten her to the ER. He had slept on a cot for eleven nights. He had taken care of her **picc line** (peripherally inserted central catheter), inserted in her arm for six weeks. He had to inject the antibiotics and then clean the line out with saline.

He had saved her life.

Four years later, Jake and Karli got married on the first

day of May at the beautiful Clos La Chance winery near Morgan Hill. Everyone cried— Mom, Dad, Jake, Karli, all the bridesmaids, and half the wedding guests.

Without Jake as Karli's protector, their wedding never would've happened.

The yawning position is good for resting hips, and a bottle of pinot noir is good for toasting to the couple's highest priority—health.

Sophie's Choices

Sophie's mom had her hypnotized at the age of thirteen to lose weight. When that didn't work, her mom put her on amphetamines. Sophie became as skinny as the other California girls but was a nervous wreck. She didn't sleep much, taking those little white crosses for almost nine years. Then she graduated to cocaine and sold enough to pay for her own stash. That all ended when a customer in the East Bay held a gun to her and robbed her.

"I never sold drugs again," she said.

Sophie moved to Sebastopol when she was twenty-one. She was making candles in her shack in an apple orchard. She left the wax on the stove and ran across the road to visit her neighbor, the tie-dying woman who was crushing on her. After rebuffing the neighbor's advances, Sophie returned home to find her pot of wax in flames. She threw water on it, and the wax exploded all over the kitchen. Sophie ran for the door and slipped on the boiling wax, which soaked into her jeans.

The paramedics had to cut her pants off and took some burned skin with the cloth. The doctors pumped her up on morphine and discharged her from a Santa Rosa hospital because she had no insurance. Her parents drove up to get her, wrapped her carefully, and drove her down to John Muir Hospital in Walnut Creek, where she spent the next six weeks. The doctors shaved a layer of skin from her buttocks and cut it lattice style, then stretched it open and wrapped it around her leg. She still has the basket-weave scar up and down her left thigh and calf.

"Men don't care about that," Sophie said.

Sophie has also had a facelift, a tummy tuck, a hip replacement, rotator cuff surgery, and a hysterectomy. The hysterectomy was the biggest bummer with a six-week recovery period of no congress of any kind. To keep her new guy interested, she gave him congress of the crow. Six weeks without any two-way congress is a long time with a new guy, but Chad stuck around and is now living with her—sort of. She lives in her big house, and he rents out her back cottage. They are together when they want to be and apart when they don't.

Sophie doesn't mind a few stitches here or there.

"What's a few stitches when you almost burned yourself up making candles?"

Recovery does cramp her style a bit, because she can't be as active and vital, so that's depressing. It doesn't affect her love life much, although she couldn't lie on her side to cuddle after congress of the crow due to hip surgery, so that was annoying.

Sophie prefers to unwind with a yummy Greek wine, a red Agiorgitiko, while sitting in her wild but cared-for garden.

"My philosophy is to tap into the joy of the universe and the positive energy that pulls you through."

No Fooling Around

It was Thanksgiving weekend and Becky's second year to go to Colorado for the holiday. Her best friend, Sarah, lived in the tiny town of Saguache near the Sangre de Cristo mountains.

The real reason she was going was to see Sarah's cousin, Mike. He'd been her long-distance boyfriend for a while, and his gorgeous bearded face was calling her. Mike had broken his leg a month before, so it made sense for her to go to him, instead of the other way around.

When she got to Denver, Becky caught a ride with Mike and his sister since Mike couldn't drive. Sis drove them in his car down to Saguache for a late (next-day) Thanksgiving dinner.

Mike didn't feel good, complaining that this leg really hurt.

"You broke it," Becky said. "Of course it hurts."

Becky had never broken a bone before. But she knew something was wrong. Mike didn't smile and laugh with his cousin and was quiet during the meal. Becky didn't know half the people there, but she still had more fun than Mike did.

That night, Mike and Becky slept in the loft in Sarah and Darrell's house that they were remodeling. Mike had trouble getting up the ladder with his big cast, but he got it done. He didn't want to fool around. Becky was disappointed.

"You need to see the doctor and get checked out," she said.

"Yeah, yeah," he said in typical guy fashion.

"Promise me," she said. "Promise me that you'll go in

Monday after I'm gone."

Mike promised.

Becky tried some manual stimulation on Mike, and soon he was snoring. No romance for her.

The next day Sarah and her husband drove Becky to the forest to cut down a small Christmas tree to take back to Omaha. Mike waited in the car. He was feverish that day and sweated more than usual.

"I hope they let me take the tree on the train," Becky said.

The rest of the weekend was a blur of Becky's Chaucer homework with Mike's help. He'd had some experience with old languages before he dropped out of the seminary. Becky knew Spanish, but she'd never taken a class in Shakespeare, which is Middle English (Chaucer is Old English). She was so lost.

Becky boarded Amtrak with the little pine tree after signing a waiver that it might get damaged. Her plan was to study Chaucer on the long ride home to Omaha, but she fell asleep to the rhythm of the train going over the tracks. She woke up around 4:00 A.M. and tossed and turned for the next three hours.

When she got to Omaha, she took a cab to her apartment, where she had just enough time to change into teaching clothes and grab a cup of coffee. She went outside, where it had started to snow. She made her way to her garage and opened it up, backed out her car, and then did the dumbest thing ever. She pulled down the sectional garage door and reached for the handle in the middle section to close it. As the door was coming down, her thumb went right between the sections, and the door closed on it.

Long story short, Becky smashed and broke her thumb. She never made it to school that day. Instead, her neighbor drove her to the ER. She was docked a day of pay because the contract said anyone who called in sick after a holiday would be docked. Her nail eventually fell off. It grew back many months later, crooked and with ridges.

And about Mike's leg? He was in his second cast, and the technician who had cut off his first cast had nicked his leg. The doctor opened up the cast and found a raging infection underneath.

The doctor said two more days and Mike would've been dead. Becky was glad Mike had listened to her and gone to the doctor. No wonder he hadn't wanted to fool around!

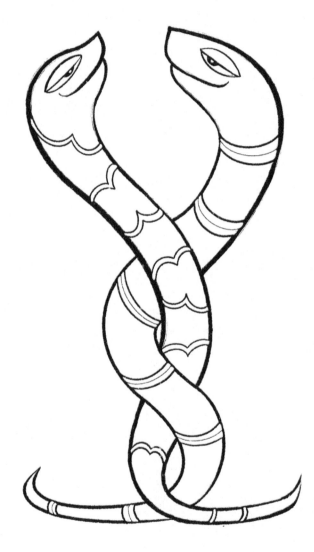

CHAPTER 13
THE C-WORD

"Cancer is a word, not a sentence."
– Anonymous

If you live long enough, you, your friends, or one of your family members will get one kind of cancer or another. But for Simone, Hattie, Henry, and Delilah, the love in their lives only got stronger.

The Nodes of March

In the spring of her sixtieth year, Simone, a lanky redheaded dynamo, was diagnosed with early-stage lymphoma, a blood cancer. Her treatment would involve chemotherapy and radiation, which would be rough but would save her life.

For Simone, the timing couldn't have been worse, as she was six months into a wonderful relationship with a new love, Rex. She had to tell him that her life—their lives—would drastically change over the next weeks and months. Having faced and conquered some hard challenges already, Simone told him that she could manage alone with supportive family and friends, if he wanted out. She would understand. Without flinching, he vowed to stick with her.

After the initial shock of hearing the word *cancer*, the next jolt for Simone was the terrifying thought of losing her hair. Imagining her head as bald as a billiard ball was more devastating to her than the cancer itself. Her hair was her thing. Who was she if she couldn't see her signature flaming mane of curly locks framing her face in the mirror each morning? How would she present to the world? Denial set in. While fully accepting the disease from the start, it was the hair-loss side effect that Simone would have no part of.

"No!" she said. "I refuse to go bald. I will be counted as one of those rare chemo cases who doesn't lose her hair."

She noticed her hair coming out at a dance. As she twirled on the floor, she spotted little tufts of ginger falling to the ground. Would people see as they crossed the dance floor? Was she the only one that noticed?

Soon it became clear this was just the beginning, and now bigger sections were coming out in her brush, on her shoulders, on the floor. Her hair came out, shedding in her wake wherever she went. Rex offered to shave her head so she could be relieved of having to deal with the agony of it going little by little. She put him off, saying she needed to line up a really good wig first.

Simone wanted a wig with hair that looked like her real hair, so she located a store twenty-five miles away that was the biggest and had the best ratings in the Bay Area. When Rex offered to go along with her, she was surprised. Romping around the huge store, they both donned wigs of different colors and styles, mugging in front of the mirror. Simone found the wig that matched her hair type and style. Then Rex got into the **boudoir** mindset and had her try on other looks, like *the blond bombshell* and *the farmer's daughter*—which would be just for them alone. Rex chose for her the blond pigtails.

Even without surgery, eight weeks of chemotherapy and radiation was just as taxing and left Simone with little energy. She felt out of touch with her body. She wasn't hungry or thirsty. Food had no taste, and her favorite chardonnay tasted like metal. She didn't want congress.

Rex was patient and loving throughout this time, content with hugs, kisses, and lots of spooning at night.

Simone's daughter said her mom smelled like chemicals.

Over the course of the next year, the detrimental effects of treatment gradually left Simone's body, and her hair began growing back along with her energy. But she didn't get rid of the wigs they had gotten that day. She and Rex could enjoy any Kama Sutra offerings they wanted, either as a ginger bombshell drinking a Spanish Rioja, or Ingrid, the farmer's daughter sipping Prosecco, or just Simone toasting with a Cote de Rhone and her own soft auburn hair, curlier than ever, now that it had come back.

Deep Throat Follies

A couple of years after Delilah's oophorectomy (see female chapter) she was diagnosed with thyroid cancer after she had recovered from her ovarian surgery.

"It sounded really scary," Delilah said.

Her doctor assured her that the cancer was contained within the butterfly-shaped organ, one that wrapped around her throat. It hadn't metastasized.

The doctor explained that treatment for thyroid cancer isn't surgery or chemotherapy. Instead, he would give her a single radioactive pill to be taken one time only.

The thyroid gland collects all the iodine in the blood, so once the radioactive iodine gets in the bloodstream, it destroys the cancer cells, with little effect on the rest of the body.

As Nurse Ratched handed her the lead-wrapped radiation pill, she directed Delilah to exit to the parking lot, get in her car, take the pill, and drive straight home.

"Don't go shopping or to the grocery store or anywhere else where people will be close by," Nurse Ratched said. "You'll be radioactive."

While the thyroid was nowhere near the pelvis area, as the ovaries are, it had everything to do with how Delilah related with her partner, Kat.

Delilah was required to stay at least ten feet away from Kit for twenty-four hours.

Rather than enjoy a loving Kama Sutra-inspired afterglow together with her partner, Delilah had to glow it alone in the spare bedroom. Once she was no longer glowing, they split a bottle of Petite Syrah. In the mean-time, it was **absentee congress.**

Cancer Between Lovers

Hattie stood in front of a mirror, looking at her breasts one last time before her mastectomy. She had cancer in the left one, and Dr. Hershel wanted to remove it right away.

Hattie's boyfriend had been diagnosed three months earlier with mesothelioma, the lung cancer one gets from asbestos poisoning. He'd flown from Florida to California to rest and to be with her, and he was there when Hattie got her bad news.

Henry stayed at the hospital room right after surgery. Hattie's nineteen-year-old daughter, Rosie, was annoyed. She wanted to be the one to take care of her mother, not the new boyfriend. But Hattie wanted them both there in her room.

Henry spent the night in the combo chair/pull-out bed. Hattie didn't sleep a wink since he was first noisy bustling around the room, and then noisy snoring like a drunken bear. At 7:00 A.M., Hattie was exhausted as Henry snored on, and the wall phone in the room rang and rang. Hattie couldn't move to answer it, Henry wouldn't wake up, and finally a nurse came in, grabbed the phone, and glanced in his direction.

"He's a lot of help," she said as she turned on the heel of her sensible shoes and was gone.

Henry may have been no help that day, but he did help Hattie get through the horrible stages of chemotherapy. The doctors attached a port above her right breast, where it would stay for the next four months. It would prevent Hattie from having to deal with collapsed veins and trouble getting the IV into her arm.

The nausea was Hattie's second horror, the hair loss the third. She had to wear weird snap-up pajamas because her arm was too sore to put on the regular kind.

Hattie endured eight chemo sessions. Each time she asked a different girlfriend to come sit with her. Henry was upset at first, but Hattie insisted she needed her **fema-therapy**. Tina came, and Terri and Stephanie and Nancy. They'd all been through it. Then Susan and Ellen and Laurie came. They hadn't been through it. Each friend sat, talked, and laughed to get Hattie's mind off of the poison going into her veins. For the last appointment, on Christmas Eve, Hattie had her two children come with her. She told them the best Christmas gift of all was no more chemo treatments.

At home, after the first chemo treatment, Henry made chicken broth for Hattie to eat. She wasn't hungry and didn't want it, but he got her to drink some.

On the second day, when Hattie wasn't hungry for broth, Henry asked what he could add to it.

"Just one thing," he said. "Anything you want."

"How about some mushrooms?" Hattie said.

He did, and she ate them. On the third day after her chemo treatment, Henry added a second ingredient, anything Hattie wanted.

"How about carrots?" she said.

On the fourth day after chemo treatment, Henry added one more ingredient. Hattie wanted noodles.

On the fifth day after the chemo treatment, Hattie felt better. She hadn't been hungry, but because of Henry she had managed to eat four days of her ever-thickening soup.

Hattie taught English at a community college. She taught three classes in a row, and one of them was up four flights of stairs. She asked her dean to change her classroom since she didn't have the strength to make it up the stairs.

Henry showed up between classes with pieces of fruit for her to eat. The students weren't sure who the fruit man was, and she never told them.

"It wasn't their business," she said.

Hattie was worried about what to wear while teaching. She'd had a temporary implant installed where her real breast had been, to keep the skin stretched out for the eventual permanent implant. The temporary breast was higher than the real breast. Could the students see that? Did they know she'd had a mastectomy?

Hattie needed daily shots in her thigh to bolster her weakened immune system. She didn't want to inject herself, so Henry did it for her. Finally, Henry had to go to Maryland to get his own chemo treatments. He left in January, and he asked Hattie's good friend a favor. On Valentine's Day, Hattie's friend, Doug, showed up on her doorstep with a dozen red roses that Henry had him buy for her since he was so far away.

Henry underwent lung surgery in March, one full year after his diagnosis. Hattie took a leave of absence from school and flew to New York to be with him while he recovered those first few days. Things went well, so she returned to California to work.

Then she got the call. Henry had fallen on a New York City sidewalk, and a Good Samaritan had gotten him to the hospital. Henry was still unconscious. Hattie got back on a plane to New York.

For seventeen days Hattie sat by Henry's side and dealt with all the doctors. Test after test showed little to no brain activity. Hattie stayed positive while her girlfriends in California texted her, fed her cats, took in her mail, paid her bills, and forged a check for her income taxes.

On April 16th, after Henry's six children and five siblings had all come to say goodbye, Hattie finally let him go. She knew she had done all she could for the gentle man whom she had loved for five years. She called home to California and asked a girlfriend to go to her house and get Henry's social security number out of a file drawer so she could fill out the paperwork to have his body cremated.

Two months later, while Hattie was still grieving, she had genetic testing done, since two sisters had had breast cancer and one had also had ovarian cancer. The test showed a genetic predisposition for cancer (BRCA gene), so the doctors recommended that Hattie have a complete hysterectomy, including her ovaries. She agreed and did it that summer.

The next year Hattie had reconstructive surgery for the permanent breast implant. Another surgery gave her a nipple and a breast lift for the natural breast. Her breasts finally matched again! Her fifth surgery colored the nipple with a tattooing process. Her girlfriends brought champagne to celebrate.

Hattie lives in her house where she and Henry both lived while dealing with their cancers. Henry's spirit still comes around to visit. Sometimes it's a warm breeze across her face. Other times it's a soft glow in the bedroom. Hattie met a widower, whose wife died of cancer, on Our Time, a dating site for people over 50. After a long courtship, they got married, and she helped him sell his family home of thirty years and move into her house. She has been cancer free for eleven years.

Hattie's favorite memory of Henry is when she was standing in their bedroom in her snap-up nightgown right after the mastectomy and the first couple of chemo sessions.

"How do you like having a girlfriend with no hair,

lopsided breasts, and ugly pajamas?" she asked as they got into bed.

Henry answered quietly, "It's my dream."

Drink it, Already!

Colin had a doctor friend who advised him to have a colonoscopy because of his age bracket. He even mailed Colin the stuff to drink ahead of time (Magnesium Citrate), but Colin couldn't get it down. The patient skipped the procedure.

Eighteen months later, Colin flunked a **fecal hemoglobin** test where he mailed in his poop. He was advised to have a colonoscopy immediately. This time he drank the yucky stuff. His procedure showed polyps.

Colin explained that polyps look like broccoli. When they get cancerous, they grow into the intestine walls. Once the polyps are in the walls, they can spread to the lymph nodes. Then you have cancer, chemo, etc.

During a regular colonoscopy, non-cancerous polyps can be removed with no surgery. But since Colin had skipped it when smaller ones could've been removed, his polyps had grown legs. He had to have surgery of the large intestine.

Colin recovered in the pediatric ICU since the regular ICU was full. Colin said the nurses were awesome. He refused narcotics for the pain so that he could get out of there quicker.

Colin went home a day and a half later. The next day he wanted to see if the plumbing still worked, so he brought home a bottle of Grey Riesling and seduced his wife for the first time in two years. They used the pressed position. His manhood was intact. It was their last time together, since they got divorced shortly thereafter.

Colin didn't explain anything about his marriage ending, except the word *dysfunctional* came out of his mouth more than once. He will always remember the last romp with his ex-wife. He had survived colorectal cancer and surgery. Most importantly, he could still be a man.

Dancing Buddies

Tim had a girlfriend, but she didn't dance. Whenever Tim went out to hear live music in the park, he never had trouble finding dance partners. He was in his mid-sixties, a good-looking extrovert in a white t-shirt and denim shorts. He didn't stop asking women to dance until someone said yes. The fact that he had a girlfriend made him safe and harmless.

Sandy liked to dance with him even if she was a bit taller. She wasn't out there looking for a beau; she just wanted to boogie. They met up at many of the outdoor music summer venues. They even drove to a few together. The deal was that Sandy would drive since she didn't drink. Tim would pay her way into the festival, and he would buy her water or soda, whatever she wanted.

Sometimes Sandy regretted being the designated driver, because Tim spent more time drinking than he did dancing. Still, it was hard to complain when the 14-piece Michael Jackson tribute band took to the stage. They had such a great sound, and it was a beautiful Sunday afternoon in Pittsburg, California, at the Seafood and Music Festival.

When the summer season came to an end, Tim and Sandy didn't see much of each other. Tim would call to say hi, and that's when he mentioned that he had basal cell carcinoma (skin cancer) in two places and that he would be having surgery soon. He spent a lot of time outside golfing and fishing since he was retired.

"What two places?" Sandy asked.

"Well, one is on my finger," Tim said, "and the other is in a place unmentionable."

"Seriously?" Sandy said. "You can get skin cancer on that?"

"Yup. You'd better get yourself checked out," Tim said.

Sandy had a zillion moles because of summers working in the Iowa cornfields, selling books door to door for two summers, being a letter carrier for two summers for the US Post Office, and from an especially bad sunburn when she went to a Venezuela beach in January (summer south of the equator) and didn't wear a hat.

Dr. Greenberg was all business when he did Sandy's mole check. She told him about her friend and how he had skin cancer on his penis.

"I can guarantee that you won't have that," Dr. Greenberg quipped.

He didn't find any spots, but the following year, after Sandy received a notice to come in for her annual mole check, Miss Tan, the physician's assistant, found three iffy places and sent the samples out to be biopsied.

Two came back as cancerous—one was melanoma on Sandy's shin, the other a cancerous mole in her cleavage area.

Sandy and Tim are still buddies, even through the pandemic, when there was no place to dance. They have another thing in common— they've both survived skin cancer surgeries.

Tim and his girlfriend had to abstain from congress for two-plus weeks while the stitches in his penis healed. Then they got back into it, although the girlfriend didn't want to kiss with the pandemic going on.

Sandy could have had congress with stitches in her leg and her cleavage, but, alas, she had been dancing all summer with somebody else's guy, and then the pandemic. She wasn't the type to help anybody cheat on their woman. So, for her, it was more **absentee congress**.

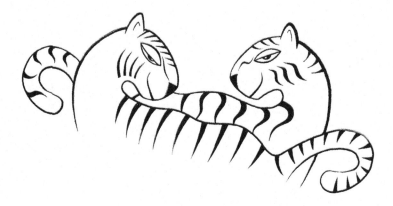

CHAPTER 14
PLASTIC SURGERY

**"Everyone needs eight hours of beauty sleep,
nine if you're ugly."**
– Betty White

Plastic surgery can be strategic for one's professional profile or as a way to be more attractive to a lover or even to oneself. When one realizes that she feels younger than she looks, she can change her reality with a snip, snip, snippety snip.

Just Take Off a Little Behind the Ears

Brenda was forty-seven when she decided to have a face-lift.

"I was in the tech world," she said. "A woman can't age in the tech world."

Brenda only told one co-worker that she was going

under the knife. She did it on a Friday before a long holiday weekend. The surgeon, Dr. Fountain, made the cuts behind her ears, peeled back the skin from her face, did his magic, replaced the skin and stretched it, sculpted off the extra, and sewed her back up.

"Don't raise your eyebrows for forty-eight hours," he said. "Your forehead wrinkles will come back if you do."

Brenda returned to work the following Monday. No one said anything, but they looked at her, wondering if she'd changed her hair or gotten new glasses. Had she tried new make-up? Something was different.

The one friend that knew what she'd done said, "You look like you've just had a really good sleep on a restful vacation."

Brenda's smarts had everything to do with her career success, but she felt that the face lift may have given her an edge with her younger cohorts. She had a demanding job but found time to date.

She met and married Max, a sexy older man who appreciated her youth and vitality. To him she was perfect, with or without the nip and tuck.

Mina's Secret

One afternoon Mina had a lunch date with a good friend she hadn't seen in a while. Seated outside in the afternoon sun, Mina's friend looked great, appearing younger and more refreshed than she had before. Chatting over a Caesar salad and Chardonnay, her friend confessed she'd had a facelift. She was willing to share the plastic surgeon's name, if Mina was interested.

"Hell yeah, if it gets this kind of result!" Mina said. "Sign me up!"

In her middle-aged reflection, Mina had spied the deepening grid of lines and wrinkles cuffing her neck, as well as the loosening of skin around her eyelids. She was dismayed about how tired and "hung-over" she appeared in photos taken when out with friends.

Mina was between boyfriends, so it was the perfect time to spirit out some of the savings she regularly set aside in her 401K for travel and leisure.

The procedure was easy. Dr. Skinner fashioned Mina a wrinkle-free neck and jaw, with eyes that looked brighter and more rested. The routine procedure involved small incisions behind each ear and across the upper and lower eyelid skin.

Mina was surprised at how little pain she felt when she woke up. The stitches were removed about a week later, and the swelling around her face and eyes subsided in a few weeks.

Fast forward six weeks to Valentine's Day. The possibility of love was in the air. Mina felt ready to attend a house party. Carpooling with a friend, she was happy to start socializing after weeks of hiding out. Upon her arrival, some of Mina's long-time male friends came up to her, commenting on how great she looked. Had she started working out? Had she lost weight?

"This surgery was worth every penny," Mina later told the luncheon girlfriend.

Two weeks later Mina spotted Ivan, whom she had already met months before through an old boyfriend. Mina flirted. They laughed, partied, and danced into the night. Ivan offered to take her home.

Mina invited Ivan in. Sitting on her couch, they got to know each other better. After some conversation, Ivan went in for the kiss. Things were going well until he wrapped his hands around Mina's face, touching her ears. The sutures behind them had been removed, but she was alarmed that Ivan would feel the scars and figure out the telltale signs of her *secret*.

"Stop!" she said. "Don't touch my ears."

Mina wiggled out of the clutch. Ivan, who thought he was making all the right moves, looked crushed.

"I just have this thing about my ears being touched," Mina fibbed. "I don't like it."

"Whoa, okay," Ivan said, "duly noted."

Mina sent Ivan home that night and didn't receive any kind of follow-up from him. She waited two weeks and then emailed him.

"No doesn't mean never!" she wrote.

Ivan invited Mina over to his place later that week for dinner. After a delicious meal he'd cooked, they settled in for a cozy evening together. She stayed over, but nothing happened.

"He didn't make a move on me at all!"

He was older, so she thought he probably needed Viagra.

"Damn, I got another old one."

After the ear episode, Ivan felt gun-shy about touching Mina. He didn't want a replay of the night they'd met. Ivan decided he'd wait for her to make the first move, but she didn't. It was a night of **absentee congress**.

After an awkward morning together, Ivan invited Mina to an afternoon Barrel Tasting at a winery. Mina loved good wine, and it was a quality pour. Mina got buzzed, and Ivan had fun. That evening went smoothly. As things progressed, Ivan put his tongue in her ear, a practice Mina said she found icky, but she didn't stop him. They spent that night together, with a successful outcome for both...without Viagra.

Given Mina's state of fitness, her position of choice was Woman acting the part of a man.

"And ear foreplay was back on the table," she said.

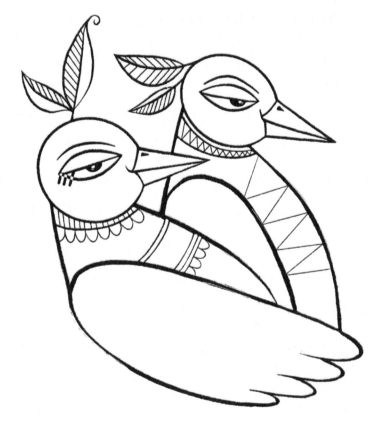

CHAPTER 15
DIGESTIVE ISSUES

**"It's been so long since I've had sex,
I've forgotten who ties up who."**
– Joan Rivers

Thomas, Lara, and PK discovered that if the gut is unhappy, it affects everything. Life is lived through the gut.

The Super Scar Turn-on

Thomas had to have exploratory surgery done due to his Crohn's disease, a digestive disorder that wreaked havoc on his body. He was cut open from sternum to groin so the doctors could take a look at his inflamed digestive tract. Thomas couldn't remember how many stitches he'd had, since it was so long ago. When his wife, Maggie, came to visit him in the hospital, all he wanted to do was have congress with her. He shouldn't have even been out of bed yet, let alone thinking about getting his horny on in the hospital bathroom. But horny won out, and when asked how he did it, Thomas remembered being really weak, too weak to even shave. He must've had supported congress, with Maggie doing the supporting.

No sinks came crashing off the wall at the Naval Regional Hospital at Camp Pendleton that day. They say hospital bathrooms are germy, and Thomas is proud to say that he contributed to the situation on that brain-foggy day. Maybe his pain meds had the side effect of an aphrodisiac, or maybe he saw Maggie as his bedside angel and he wanted to show his appreciation. We will never know, but Thomas thought congress helped speed his recovery so he could heal up and get out of there.

Thomas' new wife, Susie, reports no real Crohn's disease issues other than IBS (irritable bowel syndrome). There's nothing sexy about that, but that's no reason to stop having spontaneous supported congress against the bathroom sink with Dixie cups full of boxed wine. It might be a little cold, but think how exciting.

A Gut Feeling

Lara, a petite sales executive with a high-pressured job in a male-dominated industry, had a pain in her gut.

"I'm looking hard at early retirement because the stress of my job is migrating into my body," she said, "especially into my gut. That's where the tension settles."

Lara had been diagnosed with diverticulitis, an inflammation of pockets that can form in the lining of the intestinal tract. It caused severe pain in the lower abdomen, enough to make her double over. A mild case could be treated with antibiotics, but Lara's was more severe. The doctor recommended surgery.

After multiple episodes and months of suffering with the pain, including some midnight stints in the ER, Lara was ready to go under the knife.

Dr. Colonsky told her she would remove the problem, a twelve-inch section of Lara's lower colon.

"You won't miss it a bit," the doctor said.

There were risks of surgery, but untreated, a rupture would be catastrophic. Lara knew that firsthand. Twenty-five years earlier her father had died from a ruptured intestine, a complication of his cancer treatment.

Scared as she was, Lara decided to go for it. She trusted Dr. Colonsky.

The five-hour surgery was a success. But recovery had its share of indignities. Lara's husband, Mack, loved to take pictures to chronicle significant events. He had his iPhone at the ready to mark the occasion. Waiting outside the OR, Mack snapped a shot of his dazed wife on the gurney. Then he posted the photo on social media for all her friends and workmates to see.

With marvelous meds circulating through her system, the photo op struck Lara as delightful at the time. Mack had to answer for it later, when Lara was clear-minded enough to learn what he had done.

"I could've killed him," she said.

Four days later, Lara was discharged home, but the indignities continued. Since Mack was at work, Tex, her ex-husband and father to their two grown sons, offered to take her home. Tex had remained involved with the family after the divorce and was still included on holidays. He and

Mack had forged a comfortable connection.

Tex pulled up in his truck to collect Lara. She had to climb up into the front seat, which was difficult with stitches in her abdomen. Tex had to help boost Lara up from behind, on her behind. Indiginity #2.

Next, they had to head to her Safeway pharmacy to pick up her pain medication. Since it was an opiate, Lara had to see the pharmacist herself. Barely able to walk, she used one of those electric ride-in shopping carts provided for elderly or obese folks to shop. She had to drive through her neighborhood grocery to the pharmacy department. Indignity #3.

Then it was back to the truck, in a busy supermarket parking lot. Lara had to be boosted up from behind again by the ex, Tex. Indignity #4.

Lara was so ready to get home, but it was a challenge for a post-surgery body, especially the stairs. Lara parked herself on the main level, on the cushy sectional just steps from the kitchen and bathroom. She slept there for a month while Mack sprawled his six-foot, three-inch body across their bed downstairs.

When they were able to sleep in the same bed again, Mack and Lara remained careful not to bump the stitches. There were internal stitches as well that had to heal. The twining position was just the right ticket for the couple.

After recovery, more modes of affection were available to them. Though Lara quipped that any attempt by her husband to participate in United Congress or Congress of a Herd of Cows would launch him straight out the door, the possibility of the clasping position was on the table.

After all, they were used to being intermingled on the huge sectional while watching their favorite rom-com.

Timing is Everything

PK lived in Jersey when her high school friend's mum was terminally ill in Boston, where she grew up. When her friend called to say that her mother had died, PK woke up the next day and decided to go to the funeral and surprise her friend. She was feeling bad but thought it was the heat. She loaded up her three-year-old daughter and took off for the Jersey Turnpike.

For lunch PK stopped at McDonald's, since her daughter liked the chicken nuggets. PK never ate there, but that day she had a Big Mac. Then she felt worse. The E. coli scare was going on right about then, so she blamed her bad feeling on the food.

That evening PK got to her brother's house near Boston and went straight to bed. The next morning, she woke up feeling worse. She tried to shower for the funeral but realized she was too sick to go. Her brother's three young children and her own daughter kept coming into the bedroom as she lay there. She'd open her eyes and see four tiny faces lined up alongside the bed, staring at her.

On Saturday night, PK's brother took her to the ER in Gloucester. They got caught in a Festival of Saints traffic jam. At the hospital, the ER was filled with drunks.

"I'm in a lot more pain than he is," PK said, pointing to a guy across the waiting room.

"It's all about you, isn't it?" her brother teased.

When PK was finally seen, the ER doctor suspected

appendicitis. PK was admitted to the hospital, and Sunday morning she had an emergency appendectomy. The doctor made a long vertical incision, even though she protested.

"What if I want to wear a bikini?" she asked.

"I guess you're out of luck," Dr. Slicer said.

Meanwhile her brother called PK's husband back in Jersey.

"You should come," he said.

"Well, how bad is it?" PK's husband asked. "I have Dead tickets."

The husband came the next day after he went to the Grateful Dead concert, and a year later Jerry Garcia died. The marriage died, too, but that's another story.

PK found love again decades later after she moved to California and met a guy who had just shaved off his beard for charity, in a singles' ski club.

PK should've listened to her body, skipped the funeral, and stayed home. But then her husband would've left her to go hear Jerry Garcia, and she would've had no ride to the ER.

Maybe it all worked out the way it was supposed to.

For the time being, it was absentee congress.

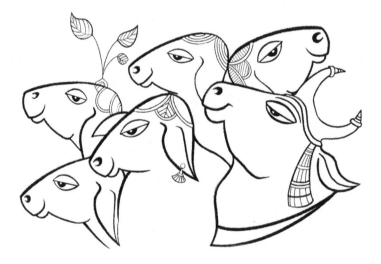

CHAPTER 16
MORE ACCIDENTS

"Sex is emotion in motion."
– Mae West

Some folks have as much empathy as a fence post. Others are there in both words and actions. It only takes one little accident to find out which one you're dating.

Gidget's Digit

One October morning, Gidget wanted to do the haunted graveyard tour in her town to learn about the settlers during the California Gold Rush, but her boyfriend, Moon Doggie, wasn't interested. He wanted to borrow her truck instead to move a hand truck to his place to relocate a couple of heavy indoor potted plants.

Gidget was happy to loan the truck but explained that she'd bought a wooden deck box for her patio cushions, and she needed help getting it out of the truck.

Moon Doggie came over that morning, talking a mile a minute about his conspiracy theory stuff, and as Gidget opened the tailgate, he kept ranting at her. He grabbed one end of the deck box, and Gidget positioned herself so that she could grab the other. Then, without any warning and still talking a mile a minute, Moon Doggie pulled the heavy box out of the truck bed before Gidget had her grip on it. The box slid down her right hand, pinning her fingers between the molded plastic handle of the deck box and the hard edge of the tailgate.

The entire neighborhood heard Gidget's scream as the plastic handle pushed into her fourth finger and ripped it open as the deck box fell onto the street. Only her grandmother's sapphire ring had stopped the box from slicing open the palm of her hand. Gidget grabbed her burning finger, and with blood squirting, she ran inside the house.

Gidget needed to get the ring off. She knew from past experience with the same finger but a different ring that if she didn't get it off now, the finger would swell up and the antique ring would have to be cut off.

She'd already cut off her great-great grandmother's diamond ring the year before. A cut from a tin can lid had become infected. She'd gone to a Christmas Eve dinner where a nurse there told her to get the ring off. The pharmacist host cut it off with the help of a stoned friend, and the MD at the party prescribed her antibiotics. Then the pharmacist gave her some samples to get her through the holiday. The ring now lived in a box in her kitchen cupboard with three wire cutter marks on the back of the shaft, and the whole shaft opened up like a pair of calipers.

Gidget stood at the kitchen sink and pulled the ring over the bloody finger. She grabbed a washcloth and wiped off the blood. The slice ran from below the top knuckle down to the base of the finger. She grabbed a towel and ran back outside.

"Take me to the hospital!" she said.

"It's not that bad," Moon Doggie said. "Let me look at it."

"Take me to the hospital now," Gidget repeated.

"Let me see it," Moon Doggie said.

Gidget held up her bloody hand, her eyes shooting daggers at him until he relented.

On the way to the hospital, Moon Doggie lectured Gidget on how the deck box debacle could've been avoided.

"You didn't tell me you weren't ready," Moon Doggie scolded.

"You didn't tell me you were going to pull it out of the truck!" she said.

"It's not that bad," he said.

"I need stitches!" she said.

The hospital was only three miles away. Still, the ride took forever as Gidget felt herself become lightheaded. She leaned on the car's window glass.

"It's not that bad," he said again. "Stop being so dramatic."

Gidget said nothing.

When they got to the hospital, Gidget jumped out of his car and headed inside. Moon Doggie shouted to her, "I have to go back to your place and get the deck box out of the street."

"Fine!" she said.

"Call me when you're done!" he shouted.

"Fine!" Gidget said again.

The emergency staff looked at the sliced wound and said, "Come right in back."

The doctor said, "You're going to need stitches."

"I know," Gidget said.

"What happened?" the doctor asked.

Gidget restrained herself. She didn't complain about her controlling boyfriend or the fact that he took no blame for the accident. She didn't tell her how the boyfriend had wanted to decide for himself whether or not she needed a trip to the ER. She didn't tell her that if she'd only gone to the graveyard haunted tour, none of this would've happened.

All she could say was, "Furniture moving accident."

When Moon Doggie came back to get her, Gidget had four stitches on the fourth finger of her right hand. He looked at the black threads sticking out of her skin and said, "Could I cook you dinner tonight?"

Moon Doggie cooked Gidget dinner for the next seven nights, until her stitches were taken out. It was his way to apologize since he couldn't form the words and get them out of his mouth. He never again asked to borrow her truck. Gidget reported that congress was okay, maybe even great. She was pretty sure that Moon Doggie has his own copy of The Kama Sutra, although now he's her ex, so it would be awkward to ask.

But Gidget couldn't get her stitches wet, so she was grumpy because she couldn't wash her hair for a week. Moon Doggie offered to wash it for her, but Gidget said no. He might have decided to cut it off when he couldn't get the tangles out.

Her Bruises, His Bruised Ego

When you ask Camille what surgery impacted her love life the most, the active single gal said it wasn't surgery, per se, but rather an accident during her solo trip to Greece.

Camille was on Day Three of her glorious journey through Mykonos and Santorini. While Greece may conjure up images of a sparkling blue sea, or a romantic rendezvous with a steamy, dark-haired local met on the boat ride from Athens, her dream lover wasn't there in Greece but instead waiting for her back home in Northern California.

Camille had recently fallen in love with Trey, a stand-up comedian. His natural humor and hilarious take on daily life attracted her to him. Within a few months of dating bliss, they decided to move in together, but the timing couldn't have been worse. Being an independent woman accustomed to taking trips abroad by herself, she had booked her vacation to Greece well in advance.

Camille was not going to let the new boyfriend hinder her plan, no matter how much she loved him. She boarded her flight hours after his shirts were unpacked and hung up in her (now their) closet and underwear and socks were neatly stacked into her (now his) bureau drawers. Trey agreed to bide his time alone in his new digs until Camille returned and they could begin their life together.

While exploring the small island of Mykonos, Camille made a decision that would change up any grand homecoming plans they had made. She loved motorcycles, and when she saw the opportunity to get around the island on a moped, she jumped at the chance. Zipping up and down the hills on narrow gravel-topped roads, she rounded a sharp curve in the road. A tour bus was coming at her! To her right was a steep drop off down to the Aegean Sea, hundreds of feet below. Camille braked hard, causing the rear tire to slide out from under her, and the moped went down. She skidded across the gravel on her side.

Amazingly, Camille avoided both the bus and the cliff edge. She was banged up, but nothing seemed broken. After getting her wits about her, she dusted herself off, climbed on the moped, and maneuvered back to her hotel.

"It even hurt to breathe," she remembered.

In her hotel room, Camille stripped and discovered a deep bruise spreading along the left side of her body extending from shoulder to ankle.

"OMG, I looked like an eggplant!"

Getting through the rest of her trip pain-free meant lots of self-medicating with **Ouzo**, a wonder tonic readily available on the island. Through the long flight home and liberal splashes of vodka which replaced Ouzo as her pain-reliever of choice, Camille looked forward to climbing into bed to heal.

"It hurt to be touched," she said.

Trey, who had been anticipating their intimate reunion, faced the fact that he had to wait a while longer to enjoy congress with his lovely lady. But that didn't dampen his famous sense of humor. Every time they talked, he would inevitably crack her up, which rattled her sore insides. It seems like laughter-is-the-best-medicine wisdom didn't ring true in this case.

The only Kama Sutra position that was possible for Camille during her recovery was giving congress of the crow, which turned out to be a pretty good deal for Trey after all.

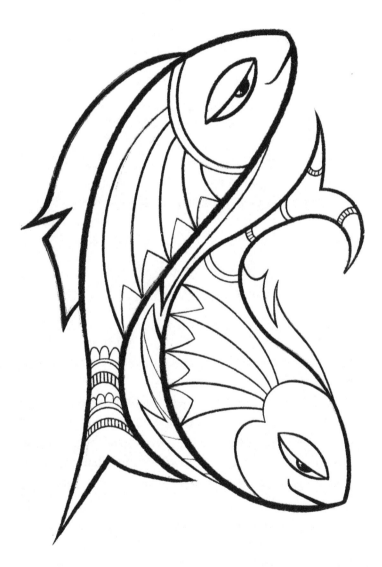

CHAPTER 17
THE BIG O

"I'll have what she's having."
– Estelle Reiner from "When Harry Met Sally"

Some of us figured it out as kids in too-tight hand-me-downs. If not, a myriad of books and videos are out there. Seek and ye shall find.

For the women who have never had the pleasure of the big O, maybe it's time to suggest to your partner that you'd like to switch things up and try a new position or two. Do you own a copy of Kama Sutra? It's available online for only $3.95 (and free shipping on orders over $35.00). Buy nine copies and give them out as gifts. Then everybody wins, you get free shipping, and you get to find the position that will finally bring you to the one big O, or lots of little o's.

Vatsyayana says in the Kama Sutra, regarding emissions:

"Females do not emit as males do. The males simply remove their desire, while the females, from their consciousness of desire, feel a certain kind of pleasure, which gives them satisfaction but it is impossible for them to tell you what kind of pleasure they feel. The fact from which this becomes evident is, that males, when engaged in congress cease of themselves after emission, and are satisfied, but it is not so with females."

What a smart guy, that Vatsyayana!

We all know women who have faked orgasms. Think Meg Ryan in *When Harry Met Sally*, during the restaurant scene where Rob Reiner's mother, the older lady at the next table, tells the waiter, "I'll have what she's having!"

Our translation of modern-day emissions—

Men emit, roll over, and go to sleep.

Women emit again and again (those lucky enough to have partners who try lots of positions until they get it right), or not at all (those who have partners who do the same old, same old).

Wake up, gentlemen, it's a whole new world out there with twenty-six positions to guide you. Don't let surgery bring you down (bring anything down!).

Scars be damned!

Wrinkles be damned!

All that matters is that the yoni and lingham meet and greet 'til things are sweet.

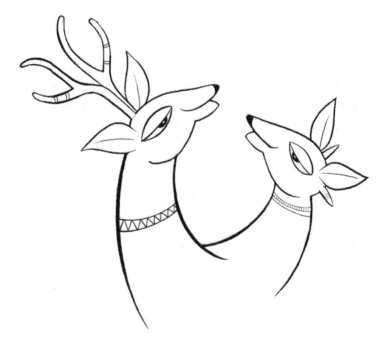

CHAPTER 18
THE NEVER-HAVE-HADS

"When it comes to sex, the most important six inches
are the ones between the ears."
– Dr. Ruth

Lucky are those who have avoided injury or illness that
can get in the way of love and congress. Just remember,
sh*t happens, and your turn might be right around the
corner.

Many of our friends have never had surgery. They have no
grisly stories of torn rotator cuffs, bad knees, bum hips,
broken bones, or gory surgeries. We feel so sorry for them
that they can't be interviewed for the book. To make the
never-have-hads feel better about themselves, we have
provided some blank pages for their autographs.

Feel free to have your no-surgery friends sign your
book, as you stare blankly at one another across the coffee

shop table. There must be something else you can talk about. But beware, after they sign, they may stand up, twist their ankle on a wet napkin, and slip on the polished cement floor, going down with a bang onto their tailbone. It is Murphy's Law, after all, that once someone brags about something and puts it in writing as a never-have-hadder, life will interfere and move them over to the other column.

So, signers beware! You, too, may qualify for one of our many topic-specific sequels: KS for Weekend Warriors, KS for Armchair Quarterbacks, KS for Reduced Carbon Footprint, KS for the Housewives of Contra Costa County, etc.

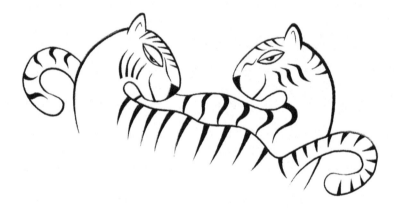

CHAPTER 19
OPTHO-PROCTO-RECTOMY

**"Honey, you're never going to get laid
until you shave that off."**
– K.J. Haypenny

This is the best surgery for moving toward a positive and love-filled life, plus there's no need to check into a hospital.

A Hairy Story

Sam raised $4000 shaving off his beard for charity. He told us about a surgery we'd never heard of, the optho-procto-rectomy. As he went on to explain it, we realized that he was into the middle of what he considered a good joke, with the punch line being, of course, that "it removes the patient's shitty attitude." Isn't what this whole book is about? If you have surgery and dwell on how old you are and how many surgeries you've had, you could talk yourself into giving up a love life forever. We are here to tell you that you don't need to do that.

Have your optho-procto-rectomy today and get on with living. Motion is lotion. Or rather, it's the motion in the ocean. At any rate, there are a whole lot of us who've had surgery and can still manage to have fun in the sack or the back seat or the tent or the hotel room. You are not alone. Thousands have recovered from what you are going through. If you keep your sense of humor about you, congress will be yours again.

FYI, the week after Sam shaved off his beard for charity, he met the love of his life. When she later saw a photo of him with the long, gray hillbilly facial hair, her comment was, "No frigging way!"

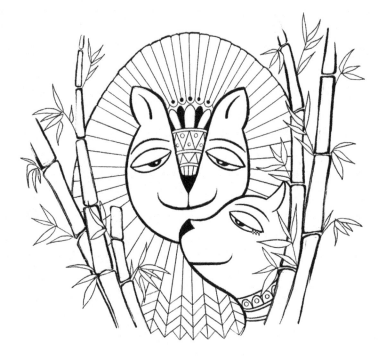

CHAPTER 20
IS THE Kama Sutra PC TODAY?

"I think it is funny that we were freer about sexuality in the 4th century B.C. It is a little disconcerting."
– Angelina Jolie

Have you read a translation of the Kama Sutra? We hadn't until we began this project. We encourage you to get a copy and refer to it as a manual, but if you don't want to, we will hit the high points for you.

Written circa 300 A.D. by Mallanaga Vatsyayana, the book still holds up in many ways. Regarding the sixty-four arts of love, family, and congress, the book states that singing, dancing, composing poetry, and culinary arts are important shared activities. It even lists tattooing, which has become more mainstream today.

As far as the term *politically correct* goes, some people have weaponized it to be a negative term. Instead of PC, let's just say *acceptable in present-day life.*

Other shared activities listed in the Kama Sutra are not acceptable in present-day life, not even close. The playing of music on glasses filled with water seems like a luxury in the drought-stricken sections of the world. Yes, Sandra Bullock did it as her talent in the film, *Miss Congeniality,* until the other thirsty contestants ruined it by drinking the water. Nowadays, when a person has to request water at a restaurant or clean sheets at a hotel, playing with water seems frivolous and unnecessary.

According to Vatsyayana, magic or sorcery is shared activity #21, but we don't think it makes for good foreplay unless you are Penn and Teller or Siegfried and Roy (Roy has died since we wrote this). The art of making parrots, flowers, tufts, tassels, bunches, or knobs out of thread sounds like a lot of work, plus you'd need your eyeglasses, and who knows where you put them?

The art of mimicry or imitation, #29, is unacceptable in present-day life in a world where everyone wants to stand out as an individual.

Practicing with a sword, single stick, quarterstaff, or bow and arrow, shared activity #32, is better left to the outdoors and is not recommended in the house, especially not in the **boudoir.**

The art of teaching parrots or starlings to speak, #42, might have been a great time-passer in 300 A.D., but nowadays, not so much. Our favorite shared activity, #59, the ability to perform gymnastics, certainly explains how followers of the Kama Sutra were able to execute some of the more complicated positions of congress.

The least politically correct of all the arts of the ancient

Indian love manual would have to be #41, the art of cock fighting, quail fighting, and ram fighting. We don't know about your lifestyles, but ours do not include blood and death for entertainment's sake.

"Honey, let's go watch two birds rip each other apart and then we'll make mad passionate love afterward."

"Yes, dear, you really know how to get my juices flowing."

Vatsyayana also stated that there are certain women who should not be enjoyed. This line alone screams political incorrectness. Enjoyment should not belong solely to the male but should be a right of women as well. After all, in 300 A.D., women belonged to harems, could not vote, could not own property, or go out in public alone. However, the women of that era had a right to pleasure as was acknowledged in the Kama Sutra, but only as long as the women were pleasing to the eye. Ugly men seemed to be okay back then. There is no mention of them having to abstain from congress.

Getting back to "women who should not be enjoyed," the Kama Sutra advises saying no to a woman who is extremely white or a woman who is extremely black. Vatsyayana, some of your words are offensive!

One has to wonder if the translator, Burton, might have embellished or taken away from the original manuscripts. Since we don't know Sanskrit, it is hard to verify.

We submit that the other women Kama Sutra says are "not to be enjoyed by men" remains acceptable in the 21st century. According to Vatsyayana, they are:

- a lunatic (we know who we are)
- a bad-smelling woman (hygiene standards? good and bad smells are subjective, right?)
- a woman who is a near relation (no kissing cousins)
- a woman who is a female friend (of your wife!)
- a wife of a relation, of a friend, a learned Brahman (an educated spiritual being), or of the king!
- a woman who is ascetic (religious/celibate)

Overall, Vatsyayana's manual still holds water on many of its teachings. The romantic role of the woman has broadened in the western world, and the four types of women of 300 A.D. have become hundreds of types of women.

The Kama Sutra states the four types as:

- the maid (virgin)
- twice married woman
- public woman
- woman resorted to for a special purpose (let your imagination run wild).

Since the Kama Sutra does not supply a list of men "not to be enjoyed" we thought we'd write our own for the 21st century. These are our words:

Men Not to Be Enjoyed
(according to the authors and a waitress we met)

- bad-smelling men (see above)
- cheapskates
- cheaters
- control freaks
- cowards
- liars
- men married to other women
- misogynists
- phonies
- players

Come to think of it, the Kama Sutra is very big about groups of four—four kinds of women, four kinds of love, four ways to kiss, four ways to embrace, four ways to lie down. When in doubt, guys and gals, do your moves, times four.

Some Inappropriate Stuff

We find these comments by Vatsyayana to be impractical and/or exclusionary.

Women That Are Loose.
Vatsyayana says:
#2 a woman who is always looking on the street
(we say she might be bored)
#18 a woman fond of enjoyments (huh?)
#38 a vulgar woman (okay, maybe this one)

Women That Are Easily Gained Over.

Vatsyayana says:

#6 a woman who looks sideways at you (we say maybe she needs her glasses)

#9 a woman who has nobody to look after her or keep her in check (excuse me?)

#15 the wife of an actor (huh?)

#28 the wife of a jeweler (please!)

#36 a dwarfish woman (so *not* cool)

#37 a deformed woman (not nice at all)

#40 a sick woman (sick women need more love, not less)

#41 an old woman (define this, please. The authors would like to know.)

On Marriage for Men

Vatsyayana says the following should be avoided:

- One who has her nostril turned up (we think maybe she's about to sneeze?).
- One who has crooked thighs (who, exactly, is measuring them?).
- One who is disfigured in any way (not cool, Mr. V).
- One whose soles and palms are always perspiring (they have drugs for that, now).
- One who has fully arrived at puberty (illegal nowadays and downright wrong on so many levels).

Stuff We Agree With

On Men's Hygiene
Vatsyayana says to:

- eat betel leaves to give fragrance to the mouth (no toothpaste until the 9th century).
- bathe daily (no brainer).
- anoint his body with oil every other day (olive oil?).
- apply a lathering substance every three days (modern soap had not been invented yet).
- shave his head and face every four days (whether he needed it or not).
- shave the rest of his body every five or ten days (early man-scaping).
- the sweat of the armpits should be removed (as true today as it was in 300 A.D.).

Men Who Generally Obtain Success with Women
Vatsyayana says:

1. men well-versed in the science of love (we say duh!).
2. men skilled in telling stories (unless you've already heard them).
3. men acquainted with women from their childhood (what about h.s. reunion hookups?).
4. men who have secured their confidences.
5. men who send presents (yes!).
6. men who talk well (duh).
7. men who do things women like (yeah, baby!).
8. men who know their weak points (our fave).
9. men who are desired by good women.

10. men who are good-looking.
11. men whose dress and manner of living are magnificent (sign us up for that).

We Agree *Some* of the Time

On Living as a Virtuous Woman
Vatsyayana says:

- treat her husband as though he were a divine being (dream on).
- she should take upon the whole care of his family (mother-in-law, every other Sunday).
- keep the whole house well cleaned (Roomba RoboVac is a present-day miracle).
- arrange flowers in various parts of the house (this doesn't require a uterus).
- make the floor smooth and polished (but not slippery).
- surround the house with a garden (we agree).
- prepare all materials for the morning, noon, and evening sacrifices (N/A).
- should revere the sanctuary of the Household Gods (N/A).
- should avoid the company of female beggars, fortune tellers, and witches (some of our BFFs).
- should always consider what her husband likes and dislikes (but knows what SHE wants, too).
- should always consider what things are good for him (we agree).

- when her husband comes home, she should get up, be ready to do whatever he may command of her, and wash his feet (get an electric foot bath, dude).
- should not go out without his consent (he should come with her, or not).
- should sit down after him, get up before him, and should never awaken him when he is asleep (this is making us angry).
- the kitchen should always look clean (*look* being the operative word).
- should always keep her body, her teeth, her hair, and everything belonging to her: tidy, sweet, and clean (of course).
- should not tell her husband's secrets (we agree, and vice versa).
- should surpass all women of her rank in her knowledge of cookery (what the? Men can't cook?).
- Vatsyayana even tells what vegetables should be planted in the garden (we vote for zucchini and cucumbers, see back matter—35 ways cucumbers are better than men).

Vatsyayana, the man, left no stone unturned. Many of his teachings still hold up across centuries and across cultures, too.

Actually, one stone remains unturned. Burton's translation of Vatsyayana's **Kama Sutra** did not mention anything regarding the LGBTQ community. Of course, lesbians, gays, bisexuals, transgenders, and queer/questioning people lived in Vatsyayana's time, but they are not referred to anywhere in the translation. Could it be that the translator, Burton, left it out to avoid the taboos of the late 1800s? We think that might be the case.

Upon further investigation, we discovered that the original KS text included the joys of same-sex relations, and gender-variant people were recognized as Third Gender or Third Nature in the literature.

According to the Kama Sutra, it was acceptable for servants to perform congress of the crow on the man of the house to get him ready for congress with a herd of cows.

We believe that Vatsyayana was really onto something when he wrote the Kama Sutra. Some of his lists are still applicable. We must agree, that when it came to describing love and lovemaking, he was the bomb.

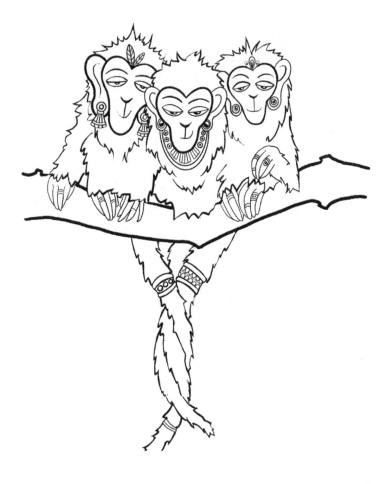

GLOSSARY OF
26 KAMA SUTRA POSITIONS

1. **Churning position** – Woman holds the lingham in her hand and turns it all around in the yoni.

2. **Clasping position** – Man and woman's legs stretched out straight out over each other.

3. **Congress of the cow** – Woman stands on hands and feet like a quadruped while man mounts her from behind like a bull.

4. **Congress of the crow** – oral sex.

5. **Congress of a herd of cows** – one man enjoys many women altogether.

6. **Crab's position** – Woman contracts her legs and places them on her stomach.

7. Fixing of a nail – Woman places her leg on top of lover's head while the other leg is stretched out.

8. Half-pressed position – Woman's leg contracted against chest—other leg is stretched out straight.

9. Lotus position – When the man and woman's shanks are placed one upon the other (criss-cross applesauce).

10. Lower congress – congress in the anus.

11. Mare's position – Woman forcibly holds lover's lingham in her yoni.

12. Packed position – When the Woman's thighs are raised and placed one upon the other.

13. Pair of tongs – Woman holds lingham in her yoni, drawing it in, pressing and keeping it in her for a long time.

14. Position of Indrani – Woman places thighs with legs doubled on them upon her, man on knees in front of her.

15. Pressed position – Woman's legs contracted and held by lover to his chest.

16. Rising position – Woman raises both her thighs straight up.

17. Splitting of the bamboo – Woman places one leg on lover's shoulder, stretches the other out, then alternately switches positions of each leg.

18. Supported congress – Man and woman support themselves on each other's bodies or on a wall or pillar, having congress while standing.

19. Suspended congress – Man supports himself against a wall and the woman sits on his joined hands underneath her, arms around his neck, her thighs alongside his waist, moves herself by her feet which are touching the wall against which the man is leaning.

20. The Swing – Man holds up the middle part of his body. Woman turns around her middle part.

21. The Top – Woman turns around like a wheel during congress.

22. Twining position – Woman places a thigh across lover's thigh.

23. Turning position – When the Man during congress turns around and enjoys woman without leaving her, while she embraces him around the back.

24. United congress – Man enjoys two women at the same time.

25. Woman acting the part of a man – Man lies on his back and woman acts his part out.

26. Yawning position – Woman raises her thighs and keeps them wide apart.

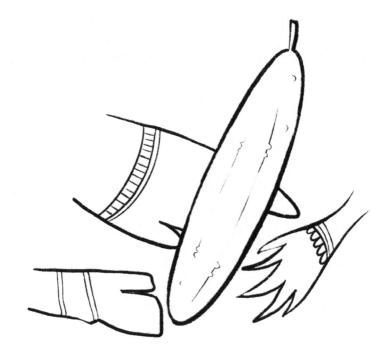

TWO GIRLS GLOSSARY

absentee congress – no sex

alopecia – loss of hair

amour – secret lover

benefits package – congress between friends with no commitment

birds in government – congress of the crow

bodice ripper – romance novel with lots of congress

brahman – an educated spiritual being (KS)

BFD – big flipping deal

bisexual – sexually attracted to both men and women

boudoir – a woman's dressing room, bedroom, or private sitting room

breech position – baby not head first in birth canal

cannula – a small tube for insertion into a body cavity or duct

Cardioversion – a medical procedure by which an abnormally fast heart rate (tachycardia) or cardiac arrhythmia is converted to a normal rhythm using electricity or drugs.

celibacy – decision to not have congress

congenital – a condition present since birth

cougar – an older woman involved with a younger man

cowgirl position – woman acting the part of a man while wearing her jaunty cowgirl hat

CPAP – machine to aid in breathing while a person with sleep apnea sleeps

criss-cross applesauce – the lotus position

deviated septum – is a condition in which the nasal septum, the bone and cartilage that divide the nasal cavity of the nose in half, is significantly off-center or crooked, making breathing difficult

diverticulitis – inflammation of a diverticulum, especially in the colon, causing pain and disturbance of bowel function

ECV – external cephalic version— flipping of a breech baby by external manipulation

emission – term for ejaculation in the Kama Sutra (not smog check term)

female supine – woman flat on her back

fema-therapy – name for chemotherapy with female friends along

Fifty Shades of Grey – wild congress, as seen in movie and read in book of the same name

friends with benefits – two friends who have congress together without being emotionally involved

FWB – friends with benefits

inguinal hernia – a protrusion of abdominal-cavity contents through the inguinal canal. Symptoms may include pain or discomfort especially with coughing, exercise, or bowel movements. Often it gets worse throughout the day and improves when lying down. A bulging area may occur that becomes larger when bearing down. Inguinal hernias occur more often on the right than the left side.

ischemic – a decrease in the blood supply to a bodily organ, tissue, or part caused by constriction or obstruction of the blood vessels

JK – just kidding

lingham – term for penis in the Kama Sutra

LOL – laugh out loud

LTR – long term relationship

Medevac – helicopter that transports an injured person to the hospital

Ménage à trois – French for congress with 3 participants

mesothelioma – cancer of the mesothelium, the tissue that covers the organs

missionary position – man and woman lie down facing one another, man on top

mouth congress – term for oral congress in the Kama Sutra

nurse with a purse – an older woman who will take care of a man with health problems and pay for everything

ouzo – anise-flavored liquor from Greece

paramour – secret lover

PMS – moodiness before a woman's period

POA – power of attorney

port – a device that is placed under the skin to provide intravenous (I.V.) access for chemotherapy, medications, and transfusions. It is made up of a small reservoir and a catheter that provides access to the larger veins. Implanted port placement is very common for patients who need long-term I.V. access.

position du jour – position of the day

roller coaster ride of irritability – PMS

Rosie Palm – slang for man having solo congress

rug rats – small children

sepsis – the presence of pathogenic organisms or their toxins in the blood and tissues, or the poisoned condition resulting from the presence of pathogens or their toxins

septic – relating to, involving, caused by, or affected with sepsis

sitz bath – a type of bath in which only the hips and buttocks are soaked in water or saline solution. Its name comes from the German verb "sitzen," **meaning** "to sit."

sleep apnea – a condition where the person stops breathing while sleeping, only to gasp himself awake to resume breathing

smudging – purifying a room with the smoke of sacred herbs

SO – significant other

sugar daddy – a man who will take care of a woman and pay for everything

sugar mama – a woman who will take care of a man and pay for everything

subservient – prepared to obey others unquestioningly

syndrome – a set of signs and symptoms that appear together and characterize a disease or medical condition

terminal – no hope for recovery

tuchis – butt

vasculitis – an inflammation of the blood vessels

vasectomy – cutting of the vas deferens, the tubes that carry sperm to the penis

Viagra – magic blue pill for male erections, also Sanskrit word for tiger

WASP – Women's Airforce Service Pilot (World War II)

WTF – what the flip?

yoni – term for vagina in the Kama Sutra

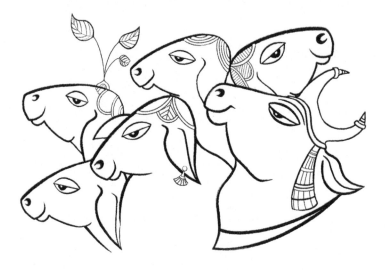

BAD BREAK-UP LINES

"It's not you, it's me."

"It's not me, it's you."

"You're really handsome, and you're quite the catch, but we work together."

"I'm not feeling it."

"I stopped feeling it a week ago."

"I forgot to tell you I'm married."

"You forgot to tell me you're married!"

BAD PICK-UP LINES

"Did it hurt when you fell from heaven?"

"Do you want to come up and see my etchings?"

"Would you like to come up for a nightcap?"

"You're one of the top five best-looking
women here tonight."

"You're the hottest chick in this place!"

"Did we go to high school together?"

"I salute you."

"Are you single? Are you psychotic?"

"You don't look old enough to wear reading glasses!"

"You know you are beautiful."

"Is that a tulip tattoo on your chest?"

"I love the Beatles!"

"My parents love the Beatles!"

FOREPLAY FOR A MAN

anything

everything

strokes to his ego

compliments

woman in stiletto shoes or boots

woman in a red dress

woman in a bikini

lingerie commercials

FOREPLAY FOR A WOMAN

compliments

dancing

hugging

kissing

man cooking her a meal

man cleaning up kitchen

man fixing her car, hanging a shelf, figuring her taxes

man making plans with her for future activities

man planning vacations with her

man paying attention to her

any or all of this in the previous six hours

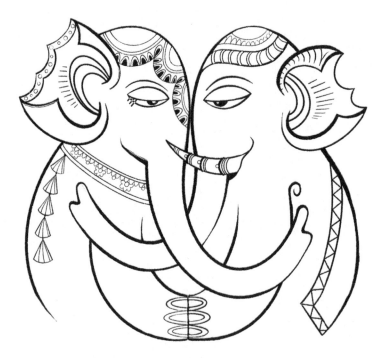

35 WAYS ROSIE PALM IS BETTER
THAN A HOT DATE

1. Rosie Palm doesn't need to be wined and dined.
2. She doesn't care what you are wearing (or not wearing).
3. She is always in the mood.
4. She doesn't look at your cell phone texts.
5. She doesn't care about your ex-girlfriends.
6. She doesn't care if you haven't brushed your teeth.
7. She doesn't care if the TV is on.
8. She doesn't mind if you haven't showered since your workout.
9. She doesn't complain about scratchy beard stubble.
10. She never talks about the kids.
11. She doesn't order the most expensive meal at the restaurant.
12. She doesn't mind if you've been out golfing all day.
13. She doesn't care if you promised to cut the grass but you haven't done it yet.
14. She doesn't bring up bad stuff you've done in the past.

15. She doesn't care that you ogled that woman at the grocery store while she was with you.
16. She doesn't mind if you call out somebody else's name.
17. What you see is what you get.
18. She knows how to time it just right.
19. She has a short-term memory.
20. She doesn't require a condom.
21. She doesn't need to spoon afterward.
22. She feels like a part of you already.
23. She is accommodating.
24. She's good at keeping secrets.
25. She will never ghost you online.
26. With Rosie, there's no risk of pregnancy.
27. She won't stalk you on Facebook.
28. She won't care if you don't claim to be in a relationship.
29. She doesn't mind sports in the background.
30. She won't bring up your mother.
31. She thinks you are just right.
32. She doesn't need romantic music.
33. She doesn't need lighted candles.
34. She doesn't need high-thread-count sheets.
35. She doesn't judge.

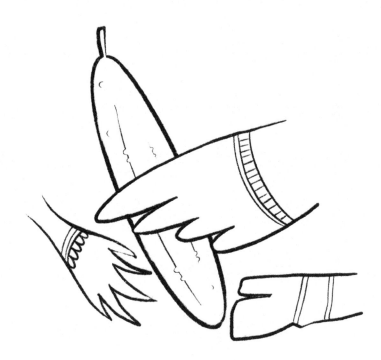

35 WAYS A CUCUMBER IS BETTER
THAN A MAN

1. The average cucumber is at least six inches long.
2. Cucumbers stay hard for a week.
3. A cucumber won't tell you size doesn't count.
4. A cucumber never suffers from performance anxiety.
5. Cucumbers can get away any weekend.
6. With a cucumber you can get a single room and won't have to check in as "Mrs. Cucumber."
7. A cucumber will always respect you in the morning.
8. If you go to the drive-in movie with a cucumber, you can stay in the front seat.
9. A cucumber won't eat all the popcorn.
10. A cucumber won't drag you out to a John Wayne Film Festival.
11. Cucumbers won't ask about your last lover or speculate about your next one.
12. A cucumber will never make a scene because there are other cucumbers in the refrigerator.

13. A cucumber won't mind hiding in the refrigerator when your mother comes over.
14. A cucumber won't pout if you have a headache.
15. A cucumber never wants to cuddle when your nails are wet.
16. Cucumbers don't fall asleep on your chest or drool on the pillow.
17. With a cucumber, you never have to say you're sorry.
18. A cucumber will never give you a hickey.
19. A cucumber won't work your crossword in ink.
20. A cucumber isn't allergic to your cat.
21. Cucumbers never answer your phone or borrow your car.
22. A cucumber won't eat all your food or drink all your liquor.
23. A cucumber doesn't turn your bathroom into a library.
24. Cucumbers won't go through your medicine chest.
25. A cucumber doesn't use your toothbrush, roll-on, or hairspray.
26. Cucumbers won't leave dirty shorts on the floor.
27. A cucumber doesn't flush the toilet while you're in the shower.
28. With a cucumber, the toilet seat is always the way you left it.
29. Cucumbers don't compare you to a centerfold.
30. Cucumbers won't tell you they liked you better with long hair.
31. Cucumbers don't care if you make more money than they do.
32. You don't have to wait for halftime to talk to your cucumber.

33. A cucumber won't leave town on New Year's Eve.
34. Cucumbers never expect you to have little cucumbers.
35. It's easy to drop a cucumber.

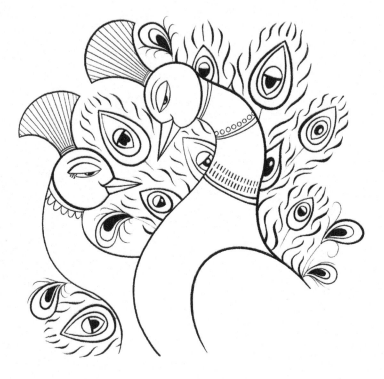

FAMOUS QUOTATIONS
AS SPOKEN OR HEARD DURING
COMMITTEE MEETINGS

"The WC Marriott is my magical place for interviews."

"Men never ask directions, and they never go back
for the follow-up exam."

"A man needs sex to give love.
A woman needs love to give sex."

"Carbonated water—it's a party in my mouth."

"Congress, it's not the kind where nothing gets done."

"Congress is a pain management strategy."

"That town is full of newlyweds and nearly-deads."

"You used to have to go to Good Vibrations in Berkeley
to buy Astroglide, but now you can buy it
at CVS with dark glasses."

"Results may vary."

"It's a placeholder relationship
until the real one comes along."

"When is the twerking Olympics?"

"Shall we draw some birds on that page?"

"Sporting of the Sparrow will cause bird confusion."

"The urge to have sex is universal."

"An older woman wants a guy who is able to hear,
who can drive after dark, and who has working knees."

"Her second time at bat came out of left field."

"Our book is about the conscious coupling of two lovers."

"United congress is not the Senate and the House!"

"That guy wants a nurse with a purse."

"You are on a punctuation diet."

"And an adverb diet."

"They sure are getting thin...those laptops."

"Have your tweezers ready, so you don't get a splinter."

BIBLIOGRAPHY

en.Wikipedia.org/wiki/kama_sutra

Fowkes, Charles, The Illustrated Kama Sutra, Park Street Press, Vermont, 1987.

The Kama Sutra of Vatsyayana: The Classic Burton Translation, Dover Publications, Inc., Mineola, New York, 2006.

Vatsyayana, Mallanaga, The Art of the Kama Sutra, Metro Books, New York, 2011.

www.sapiens.org

ACKNOWLEDGEMENTS

We'd like to thank all the folks whose stories made this book possible: Ann, Bev, Bill, Chuck, Cindy, Dan, Deana, Dennis, Don, Dot, Ellen, Gary, Janis, Joan, Juli, Karen, Kate, Katie, Laurie, Lee, Lisa, Lynn, Marc, Marcus, Margo, Marijane, Mark, Nancy, Paul, Pete, Renn, Robert, Robin, Rocky, Ron, Ruth Ann, Stephanie, Steven, Suanne, Susan, Tess, Tom, Tony, and Wayne.

ABOUT ATMOSPHERE PRESS

Atmosphere Press is an independent, full-service publisher for excellent books in all genres and for all audiences. Learn more about what we do at atmospherepress.com.

We encourage you to check out some of Atmosphere's latest releases, which are available at Amazon.com and via order from your local bookstore:

The Swing: A Muse's Memoir About Keeping the Artist Alive, by Susan Dennis

Possibilities with Parkinson's: A Fresh Look, by Dr. C

Gaining Altitude - Retirement and Beyond, by Rebecca Milliken

Just Be Honest, by Cindy Yates

Detour: Lose Your Way, Find Your Path, by S. Mariah Rose

My Place in the Spiral, by Rebecca Beardsall

My Eight Dads, by Mark Kirby

Emotional Liberation: Life Beyond Triggers and Trauma, by GuruMeher Khalsa

License to Learn: Elevating Discomfort in Service of Lifelong Learning, by Anna Switzer Ph.D.

One Warrior to Another: A Vietnam Combat Veteran's Reflection, by Richard Cleaves

Waking Up Marriage, by Bill O'Herron

Sex—Interrupted: Igniting Intimacy While Living With Illness or Disability, by Iris Zink and Jenny Palter

ABOUT THE AUTHORS

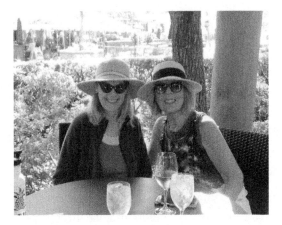

Becca Haussmann

Becca Haussmann grew up in the Midwest with a bunch of siblings, lots of relatives, and a gaggle of neighborhood friends. She didn't know how good she had it, riding bikes and walking everywhere, playing outside until the porch-lights came on, and visiting her grandparents on Sundays.

Becca went to college and had to reinvent herself and find new friends. She joined a sorority, traveled the world, and became a teacher for a decade.

She got married at thirty, had a family, got divorced, and started dancing again. She acquired a new rescue dog every time a post-divorce relationship went south. She only has two dogs, so not that bad.

Bae Bliss

Bae Bliss is a writer, therapist, and experienced field guide through the trenches of online dating for her clutch of single friends. Her interests and hobbies are diverse, from world culture to watercolors, from film noir to felines, from cooking to Kung Fu, and much, much more.

A sincere travel bug, she has visited most continents of the world, lived in two, and holds at least three renewed passports full of stamps. She always comes home to her beloved Bay Area roots and blended family, which includes two husbands (one current), six children, and nine grandchildren.